PURCHASE FOR PROFIT

Public-Private Partnerships and Canada's Public Health Care System

Since the start of the twenty-first century, Canadian provinces have increasingly begun turning to the private sector to finance and construct large-scale infrastructure projects. From a critical public policy perspective, the danger of these public-private partnerships (P3s) is that they are more than just new ways to deliver public infrastructure. They are neoliberal projects that privatize and corporatize the basis of public services.

Analysing four Canadian P3 hospital projects, Heather Whiteside argues that P3s not only fail to fulfil the promises made by their proponents but also compromise public control of health policy, outcomes, and future plans. Yet, despite these disadvantages, the use of P3s is being normalized and expanded in British Columbia and Ontario through capital planning frameworks and special government agencies that support and encourage P3 projects. Based on extensive interviews with academic experts, union representatives, provincial government decision-makers, and private sector partners, *Purchase for Profit* will be important for those studying public policy in any of the areas in which P3s are now being adopted.

(Studies in Comparative Political Economy and Public Policy)

HEATHER WHITESIDE is an assistant professor in the Department of Political Science at the University of Waterloo.

Studies in Comparative Political Economy and Public Policy

Editors: MICHAEL HOWLETT, DAVID LAYCOCK (Simon Fraser University), and STEPHEN MCBRIDE (McMaster University)

Studies in Comparative Political Economy and Public Policy is designed to showcase innovative approaches to political economy and public policy from a comparative perspective. While originating in Canada, the series will provide attractive offerings to a wide international audience, featuring studies with local, subnational, cross-national, and international empirical bases and theoretical frameworks.

Editorial Advisory Board

For a list of books published in the series, see page 205.

Purchase for Profit

Public-Private Partnerships and Canada's Public Health Care System

HEATHER WHITESIDE

UNIVERSITY OF TORONTO PRESS
Toronto Buffalo London

© University of Toronto Press 2015
Toronto Buffalo London
www.utppublishing.com
Printed in the U.S.A.

ISBN 978-1-4426-5120-3 (cloth)
ISBN 978-1-4426-2875-5 (paper)

Printed on acid-free, 100% post-consumer recycled paper with vegetable-based inks.

Library and Archives Canada Cataloguing in Publication

Whiteside, Heather, 1982–, author

Purchase for profit : public-private partnerships and Canada's public health care system /
Heather Whiteside.

(Studies in comparative political economy and public policy)
Includes bibliographical references and index.
ISBN 978-1-4426-5120-3 (bound). – ISBN 978-1-4426-2875-5 (pbk.)

1. Medical economics – Canada.   2. Medical policy – Canada.
3. Medical care – Canada.   4. Public-private sector cooperation – Canada.
I. Title.   II. Series: Studies in comparative political economy and public policy

RA410.55.C35W45 2015   362.10971   C2015-901247-3

This book has been published with the help of a grant from the Federation for
the Humanities and Social Sciences, through the Awards to Scholarly Publications
Program, using funds provided by the Social Sciences and Humanities Research
Council of Canada.

University of Toronto Press acknowledges the financial assistance to its publishing program of the Canada Council for the Arts and the Ontario Arts Council, an agency of the
Government of Ontario.

Canada Council   Conseil des Arts
for the Arts   du Canada

ONTARIO ARTS COUNCIL
CONSEIL DES ARTS DE L'ONTARIO
an Ontario government agency
un organisme du gouvernement de l'Ontario

Funded by the   Financé par le
Government   gouvernement
of Canada   du Canada

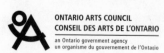

Contents

List of Acronyms

AFP	Alternative Financing and Procurement
AHA	Access Health Abbotsford
AHCC	Abbotsford Hospital and Cancer Centre
AHV	Access Health Vancouver
CAMF	Capital Asset Management Framework
CCOPS	Cabinet Committee on Privatization and SuperBuild
CUPE	Canadian Union of Public Employees
DBFO	design-build-finance-operate
FHA	Fraser Health Authority
HEU	Hospital Employees' Union
HSRC	Health Services Restructuring Commission
IHA	Interior Health Authority
IO	Infrastructure Ontario
IPFP	Infrastructure Planning, Financing, and Procurement Framework
LHIN	Local Health Integration Network
MOHLTC	Ministry of Health and Long-Term Care
NDP	New Democratic Party
NHA	Northern Health Authority
OHC	Ontario Health Coalition
OPSEU	Ontario Public Service Employees Union
P3	public-private partnership
PBC	Partnerships BC
PC	Progressive Conservative
PFI	private finance initiative
PSC	public sector comparator
REOI	request for expression of interest

RFP	request for proposals
RFQ	request for qualifications
RHA	regional health authority
RID	routinization, institutionalization, depoliticization
ROH	Royal Ottawa Hospital
ROHCG	Royal Ottawa Health Care Group
THICC	The Healthcare Infrastructure Company of Canada
VCHA	Vancouver Coastal Health Authority
VfM	value for money
VGH	Vancouver General Hospital
VIHA	Vancouver Island Health Authority
WOHC	William Osler Health Centre

PURCHASE FOR PROFIT

Public-Private Partnerships and Canada's
Public Health Care System

Introduction

Purchase for Profit

Canada is experiencing a growing infrastructure gap – a significant discrepancy between the amount being spent by all levels of government on public works and infrastructure, compared with what is actually needed for upgrading, maintaining, and developing these projects. In 2004 the deficiency in the addition, maintenance, and replacement of Canadian public infrastructure stock was estimated to be as high as $125 billion, or six to ten times greater than the rate of annual investment (TD Economics 2004, 4); this figure matched an earlier study by Mirza and Haider that pegged the infrastructure gap at $125 billion and warned it could reach $400 billion by 2020 (cited in ibid.).

Aging and inadequate infrastructure make it difficult for government to meet its social policy obligations, as the quality and characteristics of physical infrastructure (e.g., hospitals) can hold profound implications for social services (e.g., health care). The condition of, or need for, the following four Canadian hospitals in the early 2000s makes evident the range of headaches that can result.

Patients, staff, and visitors frequenting the Royal Ottawa Hospital in 2000 faced deplorable conditions for a Canadian hospital. One description at the time read, "The major buildings are 85 years old and were originally built as a tuberculosis sanatorium ... Buckets catch leaks from the pipes. It seems there are leaks everywhere ... The access to the acute-care area is by an elevator so small that when staff move furniture, they have to raise or lower it from the windows. In the treatment area itself, patients are housed three to a room. There's little privacy and they share a bathroom down the hall" (Denley 2000). At around this same time, the local hospital in Abbotsford, BC, was being described in an equally concerning fashion: "Built in the 1950s, the hospital is run-down. It's got bad plumbing, inefficient heating and wiring so anti-quated that it's sometimes difficult to power up sophisticated new hospital equipment" (Smyth 2001). Both raise serious questions about the quality of public health care services in these hospitals.

The infrastructure gap is not only fiscal. In practice its politics can include misleading the electorate. Over the course of three decades, from the early 1970s to early 2000s, residents of Brampton, Ontario, had been variously promised a new hospital or health care facility, only to have it appear and disappear in the provincial budget as the political will to fund it waxed and waned with the election cycle (Keung 2003). And in Vancouver, BC, by 2002, all but the first three floors of a fifteen-storey tower at the Vancouver General Hospital stood empty for nearly a decade rather than housing patients and providing health services as intended, all because of broken funding promises by the province (Steffenhagen 2002).

The infrastructure gap was not created overnight. It is the result of chronic underfunding and decades-long public sector (government and bureaucracy) spending restraint beginning with the onset of the neoliberal era in the early 1980s. A central characteristic of neoliberal public policy has been its emphasis on the market-based provision of goods and services in areas once collectively provided and/or financed through the welfare state. Signature features of neoliberalization thus include the implementation of privatization (e.g., the divestiture of state assets, public-private partnerships, contracting-out), fiscal austerity and other forms of spending control, regressive taxation, de/reregu-lation, and market liberalization. As a result, the majority of current Canadian public infrastructure was built during the Keynesian era in the 1950s–1970s (Mirza 2007, 5–6).

Within this vein, more recent (neoliberal-era) efforts to close the infrastructure gap in Canada increasingly centre on the use of the pub-lic-private partnership (P3) model to privately design, build, finance, and operate (DBFO) public infrastructure such as roads, highways, hospitals, schools, and water and waste-water treatment facilities. P3 can be conceptualized in a number of different ways. For Canada's longstanding proponent of P3s, the Canadian Council for Public Pri-vate Partnerships, a P3 is defined as "a cooperative venture between the public and private sectors, built on the expertise of each partner, that best meets clearly defined public needs through the appropriate allocation of resources, risks and rewards" (CCPPP n.d.). This style of conceptualization highlights the "partnership" aspect of the arrangement and downplays the privatization dimension. As will be discussed in this chapter and throughout the book, assets and responsibilities are indeed retained by the state with a P3, but many aspects of the "cooperative venture" have nonetheless been privatized – that is to say, turned into private-partner prerogatives, commodities, and revenue streams. P3 infrastructure projects are a unique form of public/private collaboration and privatization, which should be set apart from, although located within the same family as, state asset divestiture, contracting-out, and joint ventures. Distinguishing features of the P3 model include lengthy (multi-decade) lease-based bundled contracts and complex risk-sharing arrangements with for-profit private sector partners. P3s differ from full-scale privatization insofar as they are long-term lease arrangements that do not sever public sector obligations. Yet P3s are also distinct from more limited forms of alternative service delivery such as contracting-out, given that private partner decision-making is far wider in scope and duration with a P3 agreement.

P3s are an increasingly central component of the Canadian public infrastructure landscape, as is the case around the world as well. The origins of the global P3 model can be located in the emergence of the private finance initiative (PFI) in the United Kingdom in the early 1990s. In the opening years of PFI the emphasis was on the mobilization of private finance for the funding of public infrastructure and services, with ideology and budgetary pressures largely informing discourse and development (Greenaway, Salter, and Hart 2004). The United Kingdom's PFI program was quickly unrolled across all line departments and enforced by the Treasury. When the Labour government came to power following the 1997 election. "PFI" was transformed into "P3" when the emphasis shifted towards "partnerships" with the private sector. Thus the policy was no longer conceptualized mainly in terms of leveraging the financial resources of private investors, as it became more overtly geared towards fostering a reorientation of the public sector through the inclusion of private decision-making within the heart of public policy development. By 2012 the United Kingdom had nearly 700 operational PFI projects (National Audit Office 2012).

Within a few short years of PFI initiation in the United Kingdom, Canada had begun developing its own P3s in the mid-1990s. P3 use has proceeded unabated ever since, albeit in comparatively smaller numbers. All levels of government have used P3s, with some 200 infrastructure projects having been developed over the past two decades (McKenna 2012). Health sector infrastructure has been targeted for P3 use, in particular by the provinces of Ontario and BC, as the result of a host of factors, including provincial government commitments over the past decade to re/develop hospital infrastructure, and the subsequent institutionalization of P3 as the nearly exclusive method for large hospital projects. The first four DBFO P3 hospitals in Canada, examined in detail in chapters 5 and 6, addressed the need for new hospitals in the cities flagged above. They are BC's Abbotsford Regional Hospital and Cancer Centre and Gordon and Vancouver's Leslie Diamond Health Care Centre (at the Vancouver General Hospital); and Ontario's Brampton Civic Hospital and Royal Ottawa Hospital. These four stand as pioneering P3 hospital projects that have helped to guide the development of health sector P3 programs in BC and Ontario.

By late 2011, hospitals accounted for roughly half to three-quarters of all P3 projects in Ontario and BC respectively.[1] P3 hospitals relative to non-P3 ("traditional") hospitals are also becoming increasingly common in these particular jurisdictions. With the exception of the Peterborough Regional Health Centre in Ontario, since the early 2000s *all* new hospital projects costing in excess of $50 million have been developed using the P3 model in these provinces. In other words, private actors are now partners with exclusive ownership rights and revenue streams linked to most new hospital projects' physical infrastructure and support services in BC and Ontario.

P3 use shifts project elements out of the public sector and into the realm of for-profit provision. In contrast to "traditional" public hospitals in Canada where capital costs are covered through general taxation (provincial public sector budgeting) and design, construction, and health care support services are either provided in-house and/or contracted-out in limited and piecemeal fashion, P3s bundle these contracts and award them to (multinational) consortia for upwards of three decades. The for-profit private partner is then responsible for all or most non-clinical aspects of the project: financing, infrastructure design and construction, and support services (hard facility services and non-clinical care services) – and this broad scope of private for-profit activities characterizes Canada's first DBFO P3 hospitals in Ottawa, Abbotsford, Brampton, and Vancouver.

There can be no doubt that each project was overdue and sorely needed, but was the P3 model the ideal way of delivering this new

---

1 For up-to-date figures, see Partnerships British Columbia (n.d.); Infrastructure Ontario (n.d.).

infrastructure? This book evaluates the track record and implications of P3 use in Canada (particularly these four P3 hospitals), identifies forms of state support for the accommodation and encouragement of P3 use in the public health care sector, situates the P3 phenomenon within the wider political economy context, and highlights changes in the roles and responsibilities of state and market actors that accompany P3 use. As will be demonstrated throughout the chapters that follow, addressing the need for public infrastructure re/development through a DBFO P3 leads to higher long-run costs, disintegrated internal hospital management, a loss of democratic control, creates a more market-oriented public sector, and generates precarious conditions for labour, among other concerns. Despite the desperate need to close the infrastructure gap in this country, the P3 model produces its own set of problems and concerns, which cannot be ignored along the way.

The Political Economy Context

Political economy is not only an acknowledgment that politics and economics are interrelated; it is also a lens through which social phenomena may be analysed. As Robert Cox (1996, 87) succinctly describes it, "Theory is always *for* someone and *for* some purpose." The particular political economy lens used to contextualize the P3 phenomenon is described in chapter 1. This chapter advocates for an understanding of both the socio-political change associated with the cyclical nature of capital accumulation and the ways in which public policy change, though influenced by market dynamics, can be driven by internal contradictions as well.

P3 is, from a critical political-economy perspective, more than just a new way to deliver public infrastructure. Instead it is wrapped up with the widespread erosion of alternatives to capitalist markets and the narrowing of space that exists beyond the reach of capital. Marx and Engels (1948, 12) famously wrote that "the need of a constantly expanding market for its products chases the bourgeoisie over the entire surface of the globe. It must nestle everywhere, settle everywhere, establish connexions everywhere." Arguably accurate now more than ever, throughout the Keynesian/postwar era (in Canada at least) the expansion of the public sector and creation of a welfare state came to moderate some of the more socially destructive features of market expansion under capitalism by providing a social wage, actively intervening in the economy, and reducing market dependence (Armstrong 1977; McBride

2005; Wolfe 1977). Of course the reality of the Keynesian period cannot be adequately captured by broad generalizations, and Keynesianism should never be mistaken for socialism – the welfare state supported capital accumulation and at least in part "was designed by governments that wished to preserve the power of the ruling class" (Finkel 1977, 345) – but the postwar political economy stands in stark contrast to eras both antecedent and successive.

For the first time in Canadian history a sophisticated public sector came to provide key goods and services at low or no direct cost to the public. In most instances public provision through Crown corporations or welfare state activities filled gaps that for-profit actors were unwilling or unable to occupy, while in other rarer instances this involved supplanting capitalist markets and expropriating private assets (Whiteside 2012). By contrast, with the notable exception of primary education, prior to the 1930s public services remained scant, and state intervention often favoured joint ventures with capital or bankrolling private investors through corporate welfare (Gordon 1981; Tupper and Doern 1981). Further, along with the welfare state came relatively secure, well-paying public sector jobs (later enhanced through strong public sector unions), increasing the bargaining power of labour overall and socializing some of the burdens associated with social reproduction (shifting these burdens away from women and households).

With the onset of the neoliberal era in the 1980s, and even more so as of late, we are witnessing the reassertion of what Guest (1980) calls the "residual" state – where social security (broadly defined) is provided privately by for-profit vendors, the family, and charities. A key part of this process is the (re)commodification of public services and infrastructure, turning these spaces into sites of profit-making in novel yet customary ways. In line with trends common to all eras of capitalist development, original accumulation (Marx 1977), or what Harvey (2003) calls "accumulation by dispossession," today involves the commodification of social forms and transformation of common or public property into private property – making theft, plunder, and pillage as significant now as ever. However, there are also specifically modern dimensions to this dynamic that set it apart from pre-welfare-state market creation and expansion. The investment potential offered by spaces kept relatively separate from capital prior to the onset of neoliberalism is now being tapped through the introduction of market mechanisms. Hence the goods and services that are *still* provided by the public sector have now themselves become a site of capitalist profit-making and the dispossession of rights won by labour (and activists more broadly) through collective bargaining and the welfare state. Given that the state structure, as Mahon (1977, 169–70) summarizes, is the political manifestation of class conflict, it should not be seen as the victim of capitalist market expansion, but rather as its expression.

Never an abstract concept, the expanding rule of capital is animated through specific instances (projects), affecting individual services and staff. Understanding how privatization occurs and its implications can thus benefit from a sector-specific focus. Canada's public health care system remains one of the country's few progressive, collectively oriented, relatively generous areas of public policy, and it is ever encircled by the regressive, individualist, and austere political economy of the neoliberal era. The necessity of health care services make them an ideal target for dispossession, but this simultaneously helps to preserve strong public support for one of the few robust elements of the tattered welfare state. We must therefore be attentive to the mundane and less obvious aspects of dispossession within this sector, and how depoliticization is an important component of health care privatization.

The core of the medicare system – funding for universal health insurance (covering doctor's visits and treatment in hospital) – remains public, most nurses continue to be public sector employees, and doctors' fees are paid for by government, but other key components are now being gradually eroded. This has occurred in myriad ways, including through service delisting (narrowing the range of services covered by medicare), shifting care into the home (where medicare coverage often does not extend), introducing budget cuts and freezes (manufacturing a "sustainability" crisis), and allowing for-profit clinics to provide some surgical procedures (helping to foster two-tier health care and siphoning off doctors and nurses). The internal erosion of the public health care system also proceeds through more straightforward forms of privatization: the use of P3s for hospital infrastructure and support services, and the contracting-out of public sector jobs to for-profit companies. The great irony here is that the internal erosion of the public health care system began at nearly the same time as the 1984 Canada Health Act was introduced into law. This piece of legislation forms the bedrock of the current federal commitment to nationwide health care and enshrines principles such as reasonable access, universality, and comprehensiveness – all of which is greatly challenged by privatization, delisting, and for-profit clinics.

The depoliticization of public health care is occurring in two ways. First, social needs are made to conform to market dictates, and public sector responsibilities are met through for-profit providers. Privatization is a clear example of this form of depoliticization, given that it shifts areas of social concern away from the public sector and into the realm of capitalist accumulation. Referring to privatization as "depoliticization" should not be taken to suggest that it is an apolitical process; instead it points to the elimination/reduction of public sector (and democratic) control, decision-making, and authority over important facets of society. Privatization will always remain *inherently* political, given that the creation of exclusive rights of private property and the commodification of labour deeply affect the production, allocation, distribution, and consumption of goods and services, and thus power and well-being throughout society. Like Wood says of Marx's account of the social dimensions of power within capitalism – a mode of production is a "relationship of power" (1981, 78) and therefore capitalist private property represents "the ultimate 'privatization' of politics" (92).

A second form of depoliticization that will be described in this book relates to the transfer of decision-making within the bureaucracy from health authorities (both regional/local and provincial) to arm's-length commercialized Crown corporations designed with the express purpose of facilitating privatization (specialized government agencies charged with promoting and evaluating P3s, referred to here as P3 units). Along with this latter form comes the reorientation of public sector decision-making through new capital planning routines and protocols that favour P3s (important components of P3-enabling fields). Wider social goals such as those pertaining to health outcomes, democratic control, transparency, accountability, and service quality are often compromised along the way, as change of this sort encourages or focuses on market outcomes (including market-based conceptions of value for money and risk), partnering with unaccountable private actors, commercial confidentiality, market discipline, and the quantity/speed of services provided. The use of Crown corporations to help promote privatization and its depoliticization is also a novel development within the public sector.

Set within this overarching political economy context, the rise of the P3 model takes on far greater significance than mere procurement method or way of addressing the infrastructure gap – it both creates and reflects deeper social and political transformation. With DBFO P3s, profitable investment opportunities are expanded, services are turned into commodities, the state is restructured and roles and responsibilities redefined, labour and employment are shifted into the private sector, the "public interest" is re-conceptualized, and bureaucratic decision-making is reoriented. Understanding the P3 phenomenon thus requires examining its dialectical attributes: the process (change and transformation over time and space) and the moment (unique policies, frameworks, and projects). It also requires distinguishing rhetoric from reality: the justifications offered and inherent biases and assumptions made, compared to the actual operation of P3 projects. As Evans (2008) reminds us, often "the world is not the way they tell you it is."

In an effort to illustrate both process and moment, *purchase* holds a double meaning in the title of this book. Acting as a verb and a noun, it indicates at once both the profit-oriented nature of P3 procurement and the enhanced power awarded to for-profit actors over public infrastructure and service decision-making.

Arguments

Understanding the P3 hospital and its implications requires addressing both policy and project-specific dimensions of this phenomenon. The examination of health sector P3 policies and hospital projects in BC and Ontario in this book leads to three arguments, summarized below: (1) P3s involve unique forms of *marketization* for the public sector; (2) P3 projects are intrinsically unable to meet the promises made by proponents and carry several other negative social *consequences*; and (3) P3 policy, though rooted in normative ideological assumptions and aspirations, is now increasingly *normalized* in jurisdictions that have established P3-enabling fields over the past decade (BC and Ontario). Normalization proceeds through the routinization, institutionalization, and depoliticization of P3 use within the public health care system. Even though P3s are developed in other provinces, the presence of enabling fields in BC and Ontario set them apart and help explain why P3 use is so widespread there, relative to other jurisdictions.

Marketization

P3s contribute to the marketization of public infrastructure and services in two ways. First, through the expansion of *market rule* that flows from private-partner decision- and profit-making; and second, through the adoption of *market-like rules* by the public sector as a way of enabling P3 use.

Market rule is achieved through the dispossession of rights and customs previously enjoyed by citizens, public sector workers, stakeholders (e.g., patients, communities), and the public sector itself. There is a wide range of ways in which market rule and dispossession affect P3 hospitals. The most obvious and immediate transformation is the decades-long privatization of work historically conducted by public employees (e.g., hospital cleaning, food services, laundry, maintenance, and physical plant upkeep) which can lead to more precarious employment. Given that 70–90 per cent of total health care costs, depending on the service, are derived through labour costs (Armstrong and Armstrong 2008, 125), profit for private employers is earned mainly through reductions in wages and benefits, and changes in working conditions. Not only does this negatively affect staff but reduced labour costs can also mean cut corners, with clear implications for health services and patients. For instance, when staff are provided with less training, it can lead to lower quality or less rigorous cleaning, in turn affecting infection control and hygiene.

Consequences

Hospitals account for the largest share of total health care spending in Canada (roughly one-third) (CIHI 2012) and therefore governments may be tempted to introduce privatization as a way to reduce public expenditures. Yet greater profit-making for the private partners and contractors does not necessarily translate into lower costs for taxpayers, especially when hospital infrastructure is privately financed. P3s are often used by government to avoid upfront capital expenses and as a way to shift costs and risks away from the public sector; however, higher interest rates, hidden fees, inadequate or misleading risk transfer, and higher private-partner overhead costs all add up, producing more expensive infrastructure and services over the long run. Higher-cost P3 infrastructure also places greater pressure on the community and third-sector resources required to fund the "local share" component of these projects.

Finally, the dispossession of rights and customs surrounding public sector/bureaucratic decision-making (including democratic transparency and oversight) also occurs when P3 private providers – often large multinational corporations – come to manage, organize, and control some degree of future planning of hospital services and infrastructure. Greater market rule presents a number of contradictions for the current and future management of public hospitals such as reduced capacity for future innovation (e.g., the application of new technology and spatial design techniques) and disintegrated hospital service organization and planning. P3s create an internal bifurcation of authority when private partners manage support services and public partners manage clinical services.

Normalization

Market-like rules, the other major component of marketization with P3s, reorient public sector decision-making by adopting the logic and reasoning of capital. Market-based notions of risk and value for money reconceptualize the "public interest" and become the basis upon which P3 proliferation is encouraged. The term used in this book to describe the key policies involved in this process is a "P3-enabling field." Enabling fields in BC and Ontario are composed of the following: enabling legislation and capital planning frameworks (BC's Community Charter Act, Health Sector Partnerships Agreement Act, and Capital Asset Management Framework; Ontario's Municipal Act, Infrastructure Planning, Financing, and Procurement Framework, and Alternative Financing and Procurement model); supportive secondary reforms (BC's restructured regional health authorities, and the creation of Local Health Integration Networks in Ontario); and new forms of institutional support achieved via the activities of P3 units (Partnerships BC and Infrastructure Ontario).

Contradictions and problems produced by dispossession leave the P3 model vulnerable to crises of faith for policymakers (particularly in light of longstanding public opposition to privatization in sensitive areas like health care) and to crises induced by greater market dependence (e.g., financial market volatility). The adoption of market-like rules through P3-enabling fields cannot ultimately eliminate the pitfalls associated with P3 projects, but it does stabilize the model in tough times, makes P3 projects easier to implement, regularizes the process, and creates a bias towards privatization – hence they "enable" privatization by stealth. These initiatives furthermore constitute a "field," given that they now inform decision-making across the bureaucracy and public sector.

Enabling fields therefore create a new "common sense" that alters public sector decision-making and procurement, leading to covert yet enduring support for privatization. In other words, P3-enabling fields are highly transformative, not merely substitutes for older protocols or ways to fill in gaps that previously existed with earlier modes of P3 development. The nature of this transformation can be best described as involving three processes: routinization, institutionalization, and depoliticization (RID). RID helps to regularize this form of privatization and ensures that any changes made to P3 programs affect how P3s proceed, not whether they proceed. Ultimately, through these processes P3s become the "new traditional" way in which public infrastructure is designed, built, financed, and operated. However, the hospital P3s examined here reveal the troubling results that enabling-field normalization attempts to ignore and/or suppress: poor value for money and inadequate risk transfer, misleading claims of "on time and on budget" delivery, an erosion of service quality and working conditions, and opaque partnerships that offer little accountability and transparency for the public at large.

Chapter Review

The arguments described above are explored through the following chapters:

Chapter 1 ("The Political Economy of Privatization and Public-Private Partnerships") situates privatization and P3s within the wider political economy context of a shift towards neoliberal accumulation and state restructuring. It describes dynamics such as accumulation by dispossession and financialization and looks at how the state has rolled back, rolled out, and rolled with marketized regulatory reforms over the three decades. The unique features of P3s as privatization are also discussed.

Chapter 2 ("Partnering for Profit") examines the theory, track record, and assumptions informing P3 policy and projects. Two large sections make up the chapter: the features, promises, and reality of P3 policy and projects; and how P3s were affected by the 2008 global financial crisis. Key terms and concepts and their normative underpinnings are also elucidated: *risk transfer, off-book financing, cost savings, value for money*, and *P3 evaluation methodology*.

Chapter 3 ("Normalizing P3 Procurement") delves into the netherworld of market-oriented policy restructuring. It highlights the movement away from developing individual P3 projects to instead creating P3 programs within provincial health sectors, which has pushed P3s into being the "new traditional" way of delivering hospitals in BC and Ontario. This shift has been encouraged through the creation of P3-enabling fields, the main items of which are identified and discussed.

Chapter 4 ("P3 Procurement and the Marketization of the Public Sector") explains how enabling fields routinize, institutionalize, and depoliticize P3 development. This chapter also explores three enabling-field components in greater depth: capital planning procedures, health authority restructuring, and the creation of P3 units.

Chapters 5 ("British Columbia's Pioneering P3 Hospitals") and 6 ("Ontario's Pioneering P3 Hospitals") turn to the legacy and functioning of P3 hospitals, focusing on the trailblazers of the Canadian market: BC and Ontario's pioneering DBFO P3 hospitals – the Abbotsford and Diamond Centre projects in BC, and the Brampton and Royal Ottawa projects in Ontario. These projects are analysed in terms of the historical and political circumstances under which they were created, their economic and financial consequences, the shape of the new governance model in health care, and how social reproduction (health and health care workers) has been affected within P3 hospitals. Given that P3 hospital proliferation continues, the latter portion of each chapter looks at how more recent P3 hospitals and policies were affected by the legacy of those that came first.

The conclusion summarizes the P3 hospital track record, as illustrated in chapters 5 and 6. It then looks at how, in light of these serious problems, health sector program stabilization occurred, as well as how P3 policy was stabilized after the 2008 global financial crisis – and what this might mean for neoliberal intensification overall. The discussion is capped off with a description of alternatives, and the limits to alternatives (particularly in light of the constraints imposed by P3-enabling fields) to the P3 model in health care.

Chapter 1

The Political Economy of Privatization and Public-Private Partnerships

Privatization is a multifaceted phenomenon. Not only does it take many forms like asset divestiture, public-private partnerships (P3s), and contracting-out, it also alters the role of the state and expands the purview of the market. Understanding the dynamic nature of privatization therefore requires examining both its policy attributes and how it relates to changes (and crises) within the capitalist system. This chapter examines privatization and P3s in Canada by situating their emergence and evolution within the wider political economy context: the shift to neoliberal forms of capital accumulation and public policies over the past three decades.

Socio-political change can accompany the cyclical nature of capital accumulation. "Political change" in this broader sense results not only from government activities, as developments within capitalist markets hold important social and policy implications as well. The postwar Fordist regime of accumulation offers clear examples. Fordist-era accumulation was centred upon mass production and consumption, rising productivity and income, and profit-making linked to full capacity utilization and greater investments in mass production (Jessop and Sum 2006, 60). Fordism thus held profound social, political, and economic implications – influencing institutions, norms, and organizational forms such as the system of collective bargaining, social reproduction, the scope of the welfare state, and banking and financial arrangements. Neoliberal-era accumulation instead features dynamics such as accumulation by dispossession (e.g., privatization) and financialization (i.e., a growing influence, even dominance, of financial markets, institutions, actors, and rationale over economic policies, processes, and outcomes), which hold their own unique implications for the state, public policy, and society more generally.

Never wholly determinative, economic considerations such as market constraints and financial instability coexist with policy choice and flexibility. State restructuring is often strategic and historically specific, and rarely if ever entirely dictated by market imperatives. The range of policy options available to decision-makers becomes most obvious when state intervention is viewed from a historical perspective, and this chapter focuses on political-economic evolution within the neoliberal era (roughly 1980 to today). One predominant feature of neoliberal policy has been its emphasis on marketization: shifting what were previously public sector responsibilities into the realm of the for-profit private sector, and the subjection of policy practices and bureaucratic decision-making to market-like rules. The former expands market rule over an ever-wider array of social concerns and fosters greater market-dependence within the public sector; the latter reorients public sector decision-making and incorporates market-based reasoning into the formulation and execution of public policy.

Just as the capitalist system is inherently unstable, so too is neoliberal-era accumulation and public policy. Witnessed over the past thirty years, the failure of neoliberal-era market politics to generate sustained economic growth and widespread prosperity has led to variations within the policy mix (some incremental, some sudden) in tandem with economic turbulence over this same period – yet for all its failures, neoliberal policies have evolved rather than being abandoned. As described by Peck and Tickell (2002), in the late 1970s/early 1980s the neoliberal era was ushered in through a rolling-back of the Keynesian welfare state, but by the 1990s new practices and prescriptions began to mark a phase of neoliberal rollout. Even with the challenges presented by the 2008 global financial crisis and the discrediting of certain core tenets of the paradigm (Fine and Hall 2012, 50), neoliberalism is increasingly normalized, having largely attained the mantle of a pragmatic or "common sense" way of governing. The growing normalization of privatization and P3s within the Canadian political economy and the implications thereof are the subject of this chapter.

Spatio-Temporal Fixes and Accumulation by Dispossession

In contrast to neoclassical economic theory that views capitalist markets as "failure-free" (Pitelis 1992, 14) – relegating moments of crisis to random and exogenous events such as sudden supply shocks (e.g., changes in the price of oil), government failure (as the monetarist school would argue, see Friedman 1962), or even to microeconomic concerns such as incomplete information (Pitelis 1992) – within the heterodox political economy tradition the cyclical and crisis-prone nature of capitalism is often the primary focus of analysis. There are several leading perspectives on the underlying causes of capitalist crises, none of which can be adequately examined here (see McBride and Whiteside 2011b, chapter 2 for a more complete summary). These include long-wave theories such as those propounded by regulation theorists (e.g., Aglietta 1998; Boyer and Saillard 1995), the social structure of accumulation approach (e.g., McDonough 1999; O'Hara 1998, 2006), and over-accumulation theory (Harvey 2001, 2003, 2004). Whereas regulation theory and the social structure of accumulation approach emphasize the arrangements that lead to generalized prosperity and economic predictability (Kotz 1994, 57), over-accumulation theorists like David Harvey point to the features of the capitalist system that produce crises and lead to endemic instability.

For over-accumulation theory, periods of crises are not unique or necessarily driven by the failure of extra-economic institutions but rather by the very functioning of the capitalist mode of production and the contradictions it engenders. Moments of "crisis" therefore do not signify a collapse of the system but instead initiate the replacement of (some) problematic features of one mode by shifting to new, more successful arrangements (Harvey 2006, 241). This new plane will typically involve three elements: the penetration of capital into new spheres of activity (by reorganizing pre-existing forms of activity along capitalist lines), the creation of new social wants and needs, and a geographic expansion into new regions (241–2). In addition to geographic expansion and spatial reorganization, Harvey adds the concept of temporal displacement to account for long-term investments in physical and social infrastructure, which he terms "spatio-temporal fixes" (2001, 312–44; 2004, 64–8). He describes how this process absorbs surplus: "Temporal displacement [encourages] investment in long-term capital projects or social expenditures that defer the re-entry of current excess capital values into circulation well into the future; and spatial displacement … open[s] up new markets, new production capacities and new resources, [and new] social and labour possibilities elsewhere" (2004, 64). Temporal displacement is most often associated with the use of credit markets to defer debt repayment, a process that has assumed new heights of importance with neoliberal financialization.

Despite taking different policy forms, all types of privatization are equally spatio-temporal fixes for two reasons. First, they all provide for spatial displacement by enhancing the breadth and depth of profitable private accumulation. Second, temporal displacement is achieved by opening up investment in long-term capital projects and social services to surplus capital rather than the previous pattern of "crowding out" private investment in these areas. Privately financed P3s in particular allow for both spatial and temporal displacement through accumulation by dispossession.

Whereas Marx's *Capital* focused on profit-making through the production process (expanded reproduction), the processes of "original accumulation" identified by Marx remain ongoing features of the system, and not relics of a pre-capitalist or proto-capitalist period (Harvey 2003, 144). Dispossession, according to David Harvey, remains continually important as it devalues assets and/or strips away rights so as to create an "outside" that can then be incorporated into the circuits of capital accumulation at low, or no, cost (149). In this fashion, new spaces for capital accumulation and profit-making are opened up.

Although dispossession is by no means unique to the current era, it is especially prevalent with neoliberalism. This includes the creation of new mechanisms to enclose the commons (e.g., privatization), the creation of new markets (e.g., trading in carbon credits), and devaluation through currency speculation (Harvey 2003, 145–8). This theory is not without its detractors, the most common critique being that it is too expansive and/or not precise enough (Brenner 2006; Fine 2006; Ashman and Callinicos 2006). Brenner (2006, 100), for example, calls this a "virtual grab bag of processes" since it encompasses, among other things, the concentration of capital, transfers of assets among capitalists, the intensification of labour exploitation, and the modern day enclosure of the commons (privatization). However, given that the focus here is restricted to its explanation of motivations underlying privatization, the expansiveness of the concept need not concern us further. Considered together, neoliberalism and its penchant for dispossession are meaningful ways to explain not only the waves of public asset divestiture in the 1980s, but also the more common forms of privatization today: contracting-out and the use of P3s.

As is the case for the capitalist system more generally, privatization and financialization create contradictions for capital accumulation. Dispossession may create new markets for investment, and financialization may temporarily defer crises through an expansion of credit markets, but both have proven unable to generate the sustained growth and prosperity required for an upswing to occur. With respect to dispossession,

Arrighi, Aschoff, and Scully (2010, 411) argue that over the long run it "undermines the conditions for successful development," and Harvey (2003, 154–6) agrees that it can end up disrupting or destroying paths to expanded reproduction. One reason for this relates to the deleterious impact that privatization can have on wages and working conditions, dampening effective demand and hence profitability. Financialization, another important component of neoliberalism, also contains its share of contradictions (Fine and Hall 2012). The expansion and proliferation of financial markets has enabled significant wealth and affluence for some, but easy access to credit in concert with stagnant or declining real wages and a decades-long global economic slump (McNally 2011) also promote unsustainable levels of debt-fuelled investment and consumption, the catastrophic results of which were made clear with the 2008 financial crisis (McBride and Whiteside 2011a, 2011b).

Transformations within Neoliberalism

Neoliberalism is a political project that aims to expand private markets and thus the realm of market social relations. Market expansion is achieved in a number of ways, state restructuring and policy transformation being central among them. Neoliberal public policy typically draws on some combination of budgetary austerity, the implementation of regressive taxation, de/re-regulation, privatization, liberalization, and the adoption of free trade agreements. However, the exact nature of neoliberal reform has evolved over the past few decades, as internal contradictions have necessitated policy learning and adjustment. Work done by Peck and Tickell (2002) on the "rollback" and "rollout" stages of this process is particularly informative. They describe three phases: first, during the 1970s, neoliberalism was mainly an intellectual project and a critique of the orthodoxy at the time – Keynesian economics. Second, global stagflation and a massive run-up of public debt were used to promote a change in policy orientation that led to a paradigm shift in the 1980s under ideologically motivated governments such as the Reagan, Thatcher, and Mulroney administrations.[1] Structural adjustment policies imposed on developing-country debtors in the early 1980s contributed to the internationalization of neoliberal public policy. This phase in the

---

1 However, it could be argued that neoliberal reforms underpin the "crisis" of the Keynesian welfare state.

1980s is dubbed "rollback" neoliberalization in reference to the destruction of the Keynesian architecture through monetarism, massive budget and social spending cuts, regressive taxation, privatization (asset divestiture), and deregulation – all of which became reigning policies of the day.

By the mid-1990s further reforms, those that were internal to the public sector and bureaucracy and more pragmatic and technocratic (less overtly "political"), were used to cement the paradigm shift. For Peck and Tickell (2002) this is the "rollout," prescriptive phase of the neoliberal project and it helped to insulate the new "common sense." Rollout policies include social program reform (rather than simply program cuts), tax expenditures as the new welfare state (rather than removing all support), new forms of privatization through partnerships with the private sector (as opposed to outright asset sales), and re-regulation (rather than deregulation).

The "rollback" and "rollout" distinction demonstrates the ways in which the neoliberal project has evolved over the years, the emergence of P3s in the 1990s on the heels of full-scale privatization being a prime example. Federal privatization initiatives, ranked according to sales proceeds, include CNR (1995, $2.1 billion); Petro-Canada (1991, $1.7 billion); NavCanada (1996, $1.5 billion); and Air Canada (1988, $474 million) (McBride 2005, 103). And provincially, Alberta Government Telephones (1990, $1.7 billion); Manitoba Telephone Systems (1996, $860 million); Cameco (1991, $855 million); and Nova Scotia Power Corporation, the largest private equity transactions in Canadian history at the time (1992, $816 million) (104). Once many profitable Crown corporations were sold off by the mid-1990s, privatization initiatives switched from overt asset sales to strategies that have been labelled "privatization by stealth" (CUPE 1998; 2003). P3s and contracting-out government services have since become the premier forms of privatization in areas that are potentially unprofitable or too politically sensitive to privatize (e.g., infrastructure and support services relating to hospitals, highways, water treatment facilities, and schools).

Keil (2009) argues that a new phase of the neoliberal project has more recently emerged: rolling with an unstable, but normalized market order, which he thus dubs "roll-with-it" neoliberalization. This concept captures the normalization of neoliberal norms, mindsets, "codes of conduct," practices, social formations, and ways of governing that are modelled on the enterprise and the norm of competition (ibid.). Rolling-with neoliberalism can also involve normalization through Foucauldian governmentality techniques such as budgetary discipline, performance management, and the power of audit to discipline state managers (Dardot and Laval 2009, cited in ibid.). From a slightly different perspective, Peck (2010) proposes the concept of "roiling neoliberalization" or "failing forward," which accounts for the dominance and deepening of neoliberalism, despite its ongoing contestation.

Altogether, these accounts suggest that despite the neoliberal legacy of financial market instability, deep-rooted contradictions, and outright failure to improve the livelihood of the average citizen over the past three decades, it is, if nothing else, a highly adaptable paradigm. An important part of its success as a governance model over the past decade has been the normalization of its policy techniques, practices, and norms (Hay 2004). This provides neoliberalism with stability and longevity, despite its many failures. Yet across all phases, be they overtly normative or increasingly normalized, marketization remains a feature common to the neoliberal era. The extension of market rule and market dependence occurs in myriad ways – privatization being the leading avenue of marketization.

Marketization, Dispossession, and P3s

The issue of whether P3s are a form of public sector privatization has been subject to debate in the literature over the past decade (e.g., Hatcher 2006; Rikowski 2003; Wall and Connolly 2009; Whitfield 2005, 2006). To a certain extent this is a false debate, given that privatization itself is not a monolithic process and P3s are clearly distinct from other forms. With for-profit infrastructure and service agreements, dispossession occurs *within* the state, offering strong guarantees for profitable investment without severing public obligations (thus insulating the private partner from risk); and marketization involves not only the expansion of market rule but also market logics and norms through the adoption of market-like rules that reorient public sector decision-making and routinize, institutionalize, and depoliticize dispossession.

Marketization is a term with several different meanings. Often it is used in reference to specific New Public Management prescriptions (e.g., competitive tendering) aimed at "reinventing government" through market mechanisms that turn the public sector into the purchaser rather than provider of services (Boyne 1998; Hodge 2000; Hood 1991; Kettl 2005; Osborne and Gaebler 1992). Alternatively, the term can also be used in a more general sense, referring to larger trends of market-led social and economic restructuring (Jessop 2002; Peck 2010) or to the reduction of deep-rooted historical, political, or social dilemmas to issues with relatively simple market-based solutions (e.g., the need for greater self-reliance, consumer choice, market consumption, and/or entrepreneurial encouragement) (Prahalad 2005; for a wider discussion and critique, see Ferguson 1995). These different meanings may be equally useful overall, but in order to capture the dynamics of privatization policy in particular, marketization ought to be seen as taking two related but distinct forms. It involves both the extension of market rule and the adoption of market-like rules by the public sector. These two are bound up with processes of dispossession.

As mentioned, accumulation by dispossession leads to market expansion through the creation of new opportunities for profit-making and by redistributing assets, thereby enhancing the breadth and depth of capitalist accumulation (Harvey 2003). However, Ashman and Callinicos (2006) clarify that market expansion via privatization is not a homogeneous process, as it can involve commodification, recommodification, and/or state restructuring. Commodification turns assets that were not previously commodities into private property that can be bought and sold in capitalist markets; recommodification converts what was once produced privately but subsequently taken over by the state back into a commodity; and restructuring creates a reliance upon private for-profit provision (121–3). Achieving these outcomes (state restructuring in particular) frequently occurs through the adoption of market-like rules in the public sector that incorporate the logic, rationale, and decision-making calculus of private for-profit investors into the crafting of public policy (as mentioned above with respect to neoliberal normalization). With the P3 phenomenon both variants of marketization are present.

Market Rule

Similar to other variants of privatization (e.g., selling state assets), P3s create new markets for capital through re/commodification. Whereas traditional public works projects (physical and social infrastructure) are wholly owned and controlled by the public sector, with contracts awarded to a private company for a limited and specified role (such as the construction portion) (Hodge and Greve 2005, 64), P3s establish binding long-term contracts that allow for the private for-profit provision of public goods and services. This is reflected in Cohn's definition of P3s as "instruments for meeting the obligations of the state that are transformed so as to involve private property ownership as a key element in the operation of that instrument" (Cohn 2004, 2). Therefore, although public assets are not directly divested, P3 contracts nonetheless carve out avenues for profitable private sector investment by contractually guaranteeing future revenue streams in areas that would otherwise prove potentially unprofitable, or too politically sensitive to privatize.

From the perspective of capital, public infrastructure is now seen as a new asset class and one that is a particularly attractive investment, given its low risk nature. *Businessweek* raves, "Infrastructure is ultra-low-risk because competition is limited by a host of forces that make it difficult to build, say, a rival toll road. With captive customers, the cash flows are virtually guaranteed. The only major variables are the initial prices paid, the amount of debt used for financing, and the pace and magnitude of toll hikes – easy things for Wall Street to model" (Thornton 2007).

Major players on Wall Street (e.g., Goldman Sachs, Morgan Stanley, the Carlyle Group, and Citigroup) are now moving into infrastructure assets, with an estimated $250 billion amassed in infrastructure investment funds in 2007–8 alone (Anderson 2008). More broadly, a 2007 estimate pegged the wealth contained within the world's top thirty infrastructure funds at upwards of $500 billion – although it is almost certainly higher now (Thornton 2007). As Mark Weisdorf, head of JP Moran's infrastructure investments put it, "Ten to 20 years from now infrastructure investments could be larger than real estate" (quoted in ibid.). As natural monopolies (a status often augmented by non-competition clauses), P3 projects are low-risk assets for private investors, with captive customers and government as ultimate guarantor over the long run. Mark Florian, head of North American infrastructure banking at Goldman Sachs summarizes the eagerness of investors: "There's a lot of value trapped in public assets" (ibid).

P3s are most often structured as lease agreements and thus, unlike full-scale privatization, the state retains formal ownership of the infrastructure itself. However, as MacPherson (1978, 7) aptly describes, a lease "is not a thing but rights to the use of a thing for a limited period of time on certain conditions," and therefore *rights* to the newly created asset are actually held by the private partner for the duration of the project agreement (typically thirty to ninety-nine years). The profit motive permeates all elements of the project and its various phases of development, and market social relations are expanded throughout the lifetime of the P3. In addition, P3-induced state restructuring intensifies the dependence of the public sector upon the market by awarding authority and decision-making over the formulation and execution of vital areas of public policy to private for-profit investors.

The specific implications of dispossession via P3s can vary. Most obviously it involves the decades-long privatization of work historically conducted by public sector employees. This leads to a deterioration of wages and working conditions and thus, as Huws (2012, 64) argues, to the expropriation of rights previously won by labour. Not only does this affect the staff working for P3 private operators, but it also erodes the bargaining position of the labour movement overall, given that the public sector tends to be the principal source of union strength in a given jurisdiction. It can therefore hold negative implications for workers in general, to the extent that past struggles for universal public services are undermined in the process (64–5).

With most P3s in Canada the government becomes the purchaser of services and infrastructure, not the public, and thus the universal nature of public services may not be undermined per se. In this circumstance, as is the case with P3 hospitals, services remain universally accessible by the public but their management, organization, and some degree of future planning becomes dominated by large (often multinational) corporations driven by the profit motive, not community or competing public interests. This aspect is similar to contracting-out, although the longer time horizon and contract bundling features of P3s add a greater degree of permanence.

The financialization of public sector activities is a less obvious but relatively unique feature of P3-related dispossession. Harvey (2003, 147) explains that financialization has become an important avenue for accumulation by dispossession, given its predatory and crisis-prone nature (e.g., allowing for Ponzi schemes, asset destruction through inflation, and pension fund raiding). Privately financed P3s add to this phenomenon in three important ways.

First, under the auspices of "risk transfer," private partners assume responsibility for hypothetical project risks such as cost overruns and delays in exchange for lucrative investment opportunities (see chapter 2). Though each project is unique, investors often expect real rates of return in the 15–25 per cent range (Gaffney et al. 1999, 116; Hodge 2004, 162), making P3 arrangements an attractive investment opportunity for finance capital.

Second, equity sales can be quite lucrative. In the United Kingdom, for example, between 1992 and 2011 there were 240 P3 equity transactions valued at £10 billion, with average profit rates for private partners coming in at 50.6 per cent (Whitfield 2011, 4). The growth of second-ary markets and offshoring of PFI asset portfolios pose clear threats to democratic control and oversight, given the decision-making and influence new owners hold over the operation of a given project.

If a P3 is refinanced after it has entered the relatively low-risk opera-tional phase of the project, the private partner is often able to secure cheaper forms of debt such as bond financing rather than bank debt, which can further increase the profitability of this arrangement (see Whitfield 2010). Other leading examples of P3 refinancing include changes made to the loan repayment schedule and to the lending mar-gin, switching to/from a fixed rate of interest, and early repayment of shareholder debt. All were undertaken in the case of the Fazakerley Prison Services Limited PFI project in the United Kingdom, which increased returns to shareholders by 61 per cent (£10.7 million) over the original projected level when the project agreement was struck (UK Comptroller and Auditor General 2000, 1). Depending on the regula-tory context, often windfall profits such as these are not shared with the public partner, and the consent of the public partner may not be legally required. Loxley (2010, 69) argues that refinancing schemes affect value for money estimates conducted prior to P3 selection and "may make it difficult to ascertain risk transfer and who exactly is bearing risk and at what cost, in the evaluation phase of a P3."

Third, there is also a dimension of self-dispossession that occurs when the institutional investor that finances a P3 is a public sector pension fund. The Ontario Municipal Employees Retirement System (OMERS), Ontario Teachers' Pension Plan, and Labourers Pension Fund of Cen-tral and Eastern Canada, for example, have been involved in several Canadian P3s in the past (Loxley 2010), including the Ontario P3 hospitals examined here (see chapter 6). Entwining workers' savings (pensions) with vehicles of privatization creates a material reliance upon P3s, often involving the very same public sector workers or unions whose interests are simultaneously undermined by privatization. With this latter feature we see that short-run benefits can create long-run contradictions for those working for P3 private providers.

Market-Like Rules

The state restructuring that takes place to facilitate dispossession involves not only expanding market rule and dependence but also the adoption of market-like rules within the public sector. The reorientation of the public sector is therefore another important component of marketization, and again the P3 phenomenon stands out in this regard.

In Canadian jurisdictions most enthusiastic for P3s (BC and Ontario), P3 proliferation is encouraged through changes within government made to capital planning procedures and bureaucratic decision-making (including new legislation), and new forms of institutional support for privatization. This constellation of new arrangements can be thought of as a "P3-enabling field" (discussed more thoroughly in subsequent chapters). These provincial enabling fields normalize P3 use through the routinization, institutionalization, and depoliticization of this policy. Routinizing P3 implementation involves the creation of infrastructure planning protocols and routines that deeply embed the language and calculus of the private for-profit sector into the heart of public policy-making. Institutionalizing support for P3s has been advanced through the creation of new capital-planning procedures and public authorities, both of which create an air of permanency for this policy. Finally, depoliticization through provincial P3-enabling fields helps to obscure the normative basis of P3 use by making it appear as though privatization is merely a pragmatic decision. Depoliticization also occurs through the actual shift from public to private authority, making it both a strategy and a reality. The transformation of public policy through the market-like rules of P3-enabling fields is a novel development, despite the fact that partnerships between government and for-profit companies have, to one extent or another, been present for centuries.

By marketizing public sector decision-making processes, P3s become a unique form of privatization. In contrast, with the sale of state-owned enterprises, the responsibility of the state to provide that good or service is severed (Grimsey and Lewis 2004, 55). Contracting-out hospital support services, on the other hand, is far more limited and particular, often comparatively short-term (e.g., five years), and the needs of the public sector are identified and planned for in-house, even if they are executed by for-profit operators. The outcome of a P3 may still entail the provision of public (i.e., universal) services, but the process of developing and operating a P3 involves dispossession, commodification, and multiple forms of marketization.

P3s are a novel form of privatization that incorporate multiple forms of marketization, allowing for dispossession within especially sensitive areas of public policy that would not otherwise be suitable candidates for more overt initiatives. Within a public health care system, and one so widely cherished as the Canadian medicare system, P3s thus offer the advantage of opening up an untapped pool of potential investment sites, but this is accomplished in a relatively depoliticized, technocratic fashion. P3 hospitals are not only infrastructure projects – they are enmeshed within the social infrastructure of the Canadian public health care system. As hospitals they play a key role in facilitating and supporting the delivery of public health care and health services. The impact on health care and health services rounds out this chapter's examination of the political economy of P3s.

Dispossession and Health Care

Capitalism poses problems for health and well-being, regardless of whether accumulation by dispossession is present. As Colin Leys (2010) summarizes this contradiction, capitalism produces and relies upon inequalities, yet leading research into the social determinants of health strongly indicates that there is a connection between poverty and ill health (physical, developmental, social), with health indicators varying by income group. Income and ill health are thus inversely related to one another, and this means that those who are in greatest need of health care coverage are those who, if forced to fully rely on the market, are least likely to be able to secure adequate coverage. As one newspaper article put it, "Wealth equals health" ("'Wealth Equals Health'" 2012). In turn this can hurt capital accumulation if the overall health of workers becomes threatened. Thus by socializing the costs of health care through public insurance (which is the essence of Canada's medicare system), public health care not only improves health and well-being but also indirectly supports capital accumulation. The importance of this relationship is borne out historically, given that one of the most important factors leading to the development of medicare in Canada was the ill health experienced by factory workers and army recruits in the 1940s (Fuller 1998, 27). And insofar as P3s erode economic advantages offered by public health care systems, they will also pose a contradiction for both individual health and for capital. The notion that P3s can help as well as hinder capital dovetails with Arrighi, Aschoff, and Scully's (2010, 411) argument that over the long run accumulation by dispossession "generally undermines the conditions for successful development."

However, as Leys (2010, 15) also reminds us, health care "is an ideological construct almost as much as a material reality." The principles of public health care in Canada, namely universality and accessibility, remain in place (for a description, see Armstrong and Armstrong 2008, 30–1), but the era of neoliberal rule has meant that attempts to achieve these goals are now subsumed within a policy discourse of efficiency, sustainability, and risk transfer to the private sector, as well as the material reality of fiscal austerity and cost control. This exacerbates the tension that already exists between capitalism, health, and health care by widening inequality.

Closely linked to the conflict that exists between health and capitalism, social reproduction is also threatened by the profitability imperative. Bezanson and Luxton (2006, 3, emphasis added) provide an elaborated discussion of what constitutes social reproduction:

> The concept of social reproduction refers to the processes involved in maintaining and reproducing people, specifically the labouring population, and their labour power on a daily and generational basis ... It involves the provision of food, clothing, shelter, basic safety, and health care, along with the development and transmission of knowledge, social values, and cultural practices and the construction of individual and collective identities ... Embedded in a feminist political economy framework, social reproduction offers a basis for understanding how various institutions (such as the state, the market, the family/household, and the third sector) interact and balance power so that the work involved in the daily and generational production and maintenance of people is completed. *Social reproduction is dynamic in that most of the work involved in it can be taken up by various actors and institutions.*

Dynamism is an important emphasis here, as the practice of health care provision within the home, the community, by the private for-profit sector, and/or by the state is a social construct and historically particular, hence the importance of understanding how privatization via P3 hospitals affects social reproduction and redistributes burdens and power.

Problems posed for social reproduction were mediated to a certain extent by the development of a public health care system in Canada. Public health care meant not only universal access to medically necessary health services (delinking receipt of services from an ability to pay for them), but also greater job security and better pay for health care workers – the majority of whom are women (see Cohen and Cohen 2006, 124). State provision of health care insurance can also reduce the burden of unpaid work done in the home, although it is estimated that roughly 70 per cent of all care work in Canada is still provided in this fashion (Armstrong and Armstrong 2010, 163). Dispossession erodes this public support for social reproduction as it redistributes burdens (e.g., shifting care and financial burdens onto the individual or household), reinforces inequalities (e.g., related to gender and income), and reconfigures the dynamics of public and private authority (e.g., expanding the role and purview of the market).

When discussing authority and influence in the Canadian health care system, it is important to acknowledge that private actors have always been a feature of the system, including within the public medicare system. Doctors, for example, have typically been private providers of health care services, making their own decisions as to what is medically necessary and where their private practices are located, and they face little oversight of their expenditures (Armstrong and Armstrong 2008, 36). Similarly, hospitals in Canada have historically been run privately, though on a not-for-profit basis (e.g., by community or religious organizations). What is new, and thus constitutes a significant shift in decision-making and authority, is the integration of private for-profit decision-making into nearly all elements of a public hospital project and the introduction of the profit motive into the long-term planning, operation, and management of non-clinical services in public hospitals through P3s and contracting-out.

Hospital P3s involve many components: agreements related to land, financing, infrastructure (design, construction), equipment procurement, and the operation and management of public services. While each P3 agreement is unique, most display a complicated public/private division among project tasks. For instance: (1) the land upon which P3 hospitals are built is not fully privatized but leased; (2) private financing is used for construction purposes but not for hospital equipment (this is a task most often taken up by local communities and thus tends to rely upon efforts of the third sector); (3) design is private and subject to commercial confidentiality and proprietary knowledge laws, although public input and approval must be sought at key stages of development; and (4) clinical services are publicly funded and managed, whereas non-clinical services in P3 hospitals are publicly funded but privately managed. The range of non-clinical-care services subject to privatization has also fluctuated over time and by project, and even with P3 hospitals that do not bundle non-clinical services within the project agreement, these may be subject to contracting-out by the public health authority. Given that control, authority, and assets are shared, P3s may represent "privatization by stealth" but they are partnerships nonetheless.

The introduction of the profit motive into public hospitals can affect both health outcomes and labour. Cutting corners in order to reduce costs and increase profitability through hospital support-service privatization creates difficulties for service integration and planning (Shrybman 2007) and has been directly linked to illness and death. For example, in 2009 BC's Nanaimo Regional General Hospital developed the antibacterial-resistant super bug *C. difficile*, causing dozens to fall ill and five deaths in 2009. Though infection control is a concern in all hospitals, the BC Centre for Disease Control reports that as the result of understaffing and improper training by the private contractor, the privatized cleaning support staff made several crucial errors in their sanitization attempts, which greatly exacerbated later attempts at infection control (Leyne 2009). This supports Cohen and Cohen's (2006, 138) contention that "because of the special requirements and dangers inherent in a hospital setting, this type of cleaning requires a level of knowledge and skill that is acquired through years of on-the-job experience as well as special training. Such training is not typically offered by the private sector."

A related issue with hospital support-service privatization is the deleterious effect that this can have on the women and visible minorities who predominantly provide these services. This includes lower wages, less secure employment and predictable shifts, and an introduction of neo-Taylorist labour disciplining and monitoring techniques (see Armstrong and Armstrong 2010; Cohen and Cohen 2006). Furthermore, support services provided in hospital (such as dietary, cleaning, and linen services) have been re-conceptualized under the P3 model, and through contracting-out, as being akin to hotel services rather than unique health care–specific services. This approach is problematic, given that these services are in fact a fundamental aspect of health care provision. Support staff "ensure the cleanliness of rooms, furnishings, and equipment that are vital to infection control; they prepare and deliver meals; they dispose of garbage and bio-hazardous material; they do the laundry for patients and staff," and thus crucial areas of health care are affected, such as hygiene, nutrition, infection control, and patient care (Stinson, Pollak, and Cohen 2005, 34). Patients and staff training tend to suffer as a result.

Concluding Remarks

The relationship between crises of capital and the attendant alteration of public policy cannot be ignored, nor can the specific nature of policy change be assumed. The emergence and growing use of the P3 model in Canada must for this reason be situated within its wider political economy context: developments within the capitalist system (including crises), spatio-temporal fixes involving accumulation by dispossession and financialization, and the marketization of state policy and decision-making processes over the past thirty years.

Dispossession and marketization are particularly useful concepts when analysing neoliberal restructuring, given that privatization equally affects the public and private for-profit social realms. As a distinct form of privatization, P3s offer unique insights. With P3 procurement, for-profit infrastructure and service agreements allow for dispossession *within* the state, offering strong guarantees for profitable investment without severing public obligations (thus insulating the private partner from risk). Marketization involves not only the expansion of market rule but also market logics and norms through the adoption of market-like rules that reorient public sector decision-making and routinize, institutionalize and depoliticize dispossession. Neoliberal market expansion is thus achieved in a number of ways, with state restructuring through the introduction of market rule (i.e., privatization) and market-like rule (i.e., policy reorientation) playing key roles in this process.

Intertwined with these larger trends, privatization is transforming the health sector, particularly hospital support services, through changes in service quality and working conditions. Cost pressures associated with public health care are an increasingly vexing problem for policymakers in Canada forced to reconcile budget constraints with the enduring popularity of medicare. The P3 model is often touted as a solution to this dilemma by delivering "public" hospitals whilst generating cost savings and value for money, and transferring risk from the taxpayer to the private sector. However, as the next chapter examines, these claims lack empirical substantiation, raising additional long-run concerns related to their use within the public health care system.

Chapter 2

Partnering for Profit

Public-private partnerships can be used in all areas of public infrastruc-ture and service provision (e.g., hospitals, water and sewage facilities, bridges and highways). Infrastructure P3s involve the private sector in a variety of ways, with the most common form being the design-build-finance-operate (DBFO) model (for others, see Hodge and Greve 2005). P3s are not merely new procurement options for public infra-structure; they reflect larger changes in capital accumulation, ideology, bureaucratic processes, and public policy. As explained in the previous chapter, the wider political economy context of neoliberalism, dispos-session, and marketization has been crucial for P3 emergence. These connections are illustrated through the track record and assumptions informing P3s.

Despite their growing popularity, P3 arrangements are seldom able to reduce public sector costs, given the historically more expensive nature of private financing and the presence of the profit motive. Risk transfer, another supposed benefit of this policy, is also illusory, based more often on normative assumptions than actual results. Finally, sev-eral methodological biases inherent to the processes currently used to analyse value for money cast doubt upon the purportedly neutral selec-tion of P3s over traditional forms of public procurement.

Problems with the P3 model, in relation to cost and risk in particular, were only further compounded during the recent global financial cri-sis as private financing became more expensive and difficult to secure, leading to several project delays and cancellations across the country. In BC, for example, construction of the Port Mann bridge was delayed in 2009 when the private finance partner was unable to secure the $700 million required to finance the P3; and, around that same time, the high price of private financing led the government to finance and guarantee a greater portion of the capital costs with the Fort St John Hospital P3 project. With the onset of a new round of fiscal austerity in 2011, one might reasonably expect that this policy would have been scrapped in favour of lower-cost public procurement. Instead, as of 2010, the P3 model began flourishing once again. In Canada this is due in large part to strong government support (especially the federal government and the provinces of BC and Ontario). Renewed proliferation is particularly problematic, given that these arrangements link important public services to highly volatile global financial markets and poorer value for money leads to higher costs over the long run.

This chapter provides an overview of the P3 phenomenon in Canada by analysing the features, promises, and reality of P3 policy and projects, and by examining how P3s were affected by the global financial crisis. Key terms and concepts and their normative underpinnings are elucidated throughout, most notably: cost savings, off-book financing, risk transfer, value for money, and P3 evaluation methodology.

Justifying Public-Private Partnerships

The standard argument in support of a P3 is that it can more effectively deliver services and infrastructure when compared with traditional public methods, as it uniquely harnesses the efficiencies, innovative capacities, and (financial) resources of the private sector (Akintoye, Beck, and Hardcastle 2003, 4). Greater market dependence for the public sector is promoted largely through New Public Management (NPM) ideals that aim to transform the government and its agencies into the procurer of services rather than the provider (Edwards and Shaoul 2003, 397). With P3s in particular there is an assumption (rooted in the public choice school of thought and neo-classical economics) that partnering with the private sector will avoid the problems associated with an inherently inefficient public administration. This translates into P3s being presented as a net gain for the taxpayer: they are purportedly able to deliver value for money through lower costs over the lifetime of the project by transferring risk to the private partner who, it is believed, will operate in a more innovative, efficient, and financially prudent fashion (397–8). The three sections that follow detail the issues associated with P3 cost savings and risk-transfer arguments, and the problematic nature of value for money methodology.

Cost Savings

The cost savings argument is derived mainly through the neoclassical assumption that market competition (in this case, for the P3 contract), combined with the profit-maximizing behaviour unique to the private sector, will lead to lower overall project costs. Furthermore, given that P3 contracts have time-sensitive stipulations, it is argued that the private partner will have a built-in incentive to produce efficiencies in order to achieve a profit (Murphy 2008). Knowledge specialization, along with greater scale and scope of activities, is also said to provide private sector actors with more experience and ability to generate cost savings (especially compared to small municipal governments). As a result, the cost advantages offered by partnering relate to its unique ability to bring more cost-efficient operations and better project management skills to the project, along with an emphasis on using the most cost-effective technologies and lower wage costs (Vining and Boardman 2008, 14).

There are a number of problems with these assumptions. First, even in the case of private sector cost superiority, savings are not likely to be passed on to the public but rather absorbed by the private partner in the form of higher profit (Vining and Boardman 2008, 15). Furthermore, cost-savings arguments do not take into account social concerns produced by reducing labour costs (i.e., lower wages, more precarious working conditions) and through a relaxation of standards (e.g., hiring and training, environmental and construction standards).

P3s also tend to be more expensive than traditional projects. These increased costs typically relate to the higher interest rates paid by the private sector, but can also result from higher-than-bid construction costs, as well as the administrative and legal fees that accompany P3s. Vining and Boardman (2008, 11) have labelled the plethora of additional hidden costs associated with P3s as "transaction costs," which include contracting and negotiation costs, and formal contract agreement costs such as monitoring, renegotiation, and termination.

In the United Kingdom, where P3s first began and where P3 markets remain the most sophisticated of any, recent reports analysing the results of three decades of P3 policy foreshadow worrisome implications for Canada's increasingly widespread P3 use. Fawcett (2012) sums up the U.K. experience when he writes that "the record isn't great" and that "using private money for public investment hasn't been an unqualified success." More specifically, Graham Winch of Manchester Business School reports that "the value for money case for PPP in the public sector has yet to be proven. The benefits gained from the availability of 'extra' finance, the transfer of risk from public to private sector, and improvements in decision-making processes are too nebulous to provide any certainty that they outweigh all the known problems" (quoted in Armitstead 2012; see also Ball, Heafy, and King 2001; Shaoul 2010). Problems include, for example, that PFI private financing costs are on average 2.00–3.75 per cent higher than direct public funding (Infrastructure UK 2010), the average private-finance contract took nearly twice as long to negotiate as large conventional projects (National Audit Office 2007), and that in order to make the scheme financially viable, bed reductions have been typical with PFI hospitals – the first fourteen PFI hospitals meant an average bed reduction of 33 per cent (Pollock, Shaoul, and Vickers 2002).

In Canada, case-study evidence points to similar results (Loxley 2010; Mehra 2005). For example, in 2012 Siemiatycki found that for twenty-eight P3 projects developed in Ontario over the past decade the average cost was 16 per cent higher than it would have been with traditional public tendering (Siemiatycki and Farooqi 2012). In December 2014, Ontario's auditor general reported that for seventy-four P3 projects (in various stages of development) in that province, tangible costs like construction, financing, and legal services associated with the P3 model added an additional $8 billion when compared with what traditional project procurement would have produced (see Ontario Auditor General 2014, 197).

Cost-savings arguments are based not only on economic rationale but on political dynamics as well. For instance, cost-related justifications are often framed in terms of the political preference to avoid government debt through the use of private financing. Thus it is argued that scarce government funds are best allocated elsewhere when large capital projects can be funded through the indebtedness of private firms (Rouillard 2006, 8). In Canada this rationale is in part ideological (i.e., the perception that public debt is a sign of mismanagement) and in part practical, given the massive cuts in federal social spending experienced in the 1980s and 1990s (McBride 2005, 106–10). P3s are therefore presented as a way to deliver new infrastructure during a time of fiscal austerity.

However, the reality is that P3s cannot actually reduce the financial obligations of the state – they are able only to mask the cost of a project through the use of a cash, rather than accrual, accounting system. Prior to 2009, Canadian P3s were often recorded as operating leases rather than capital expenses, allowing governments to benefit from "off-book" infrastructure spending by accounting for a new project as an annual lease payment to a private contractor rather than as an upfront capital expense, like with traditional infrastructure (Murphy 2008, 101). Off-book financing allowed politicians to make good on election promises or win political points with the electorate by committing to public infrastructure projects whilst simultaneously deferring full repayment far into the future. With most P3 deals lasting roughly three decades, costs are stretched beyond the election cycle and even beyond the length of most public sector careers. Accounting for P3 projects as lease payments is also expedient, given the presence of balanced budget legislation, which has constrained public spending in provinces and territories across the country since the 1990s. Further, dealing with balanced budget legislation through off-book financing avoids the application of often unpopular user fees to infrastructure such as highways and bridges.

Ultimately the justifications for, and benefits derived from, off-book financing are illusory. The use of private financing is never able to reduce public sector liabilities, given that costs associated with public infrastructure and services must ultimately be repaid by the taxpayer. In some cases, project agreements even require that the state buy back the infrastructure once the project agreement expires (Auerbach et al. 2003, 5).

In 2009 this budgetary loophole was tightened with the adoption of new public sector accounting principles in Canada (known as generally accepted accounting principles or GAAP), essentially eliminating the "build now, pay later" rationale. From a global perspective, national variations in P3 accounting systems and principles remain, although there are signs of increasing harmonization (under the International Public Sector Accounting Standards Board, for example) (see Heald and Georgiou 2010).

Risk Transfer

In light of the higher costs associated with private financing, multiple transaction costs accumulated over the lifespan of a P3, and profit-oriented motivation of the private, tangible savings for the public remain elusive. Whereas cost-savings arguments were far more popular in the early days of P3s in Canada (see Loxley 2010), today the major justification adopted by proponents in favour of P3s is based on the notion of achieving value for money (VfM) by transferring project risks from the public to the private partner. Better VfM is not necessarily synonymous with lower project costs, making it a more opaque and technocratic justification for privatization. For example, Ontario's VfM methodology manual (Infrastructure Ontario 2007a) indicates that base project costs, financing costs, and ancillary costs (legal and other transactions costs) are all lower for traditional procurement and thus P3 VfM superiority is derived exclusively through risk transfer.

Value for money reports produced for recently operational P3 hospitals in Ontario indicate just how significant risk transfer is to claims of P3 VfM superiority. With the Centre for Addiction and Mental Health P3, P3 base project costs are valued at $354.8 million compared to only $235.1 million for the traditional procurement model; risk transfer makes up the entire "savings" that is achieved with a P3 (Infrastructure Ontario 2010, 6). With the Sunnybrook Health Science Centre P3, base costs are estimated at $142 million (P3) vs $129 million (traditional); when the value of risk transfer is estimated, the P3 comes in at $14.1 million under the traditional option (Infrastructure Ontario 2007c, 14). And with the North Bay Regional Health Centre P3, base costs are estimated at $551.7 million (P3) as opposed to $404.6 million (traditional); factoring in risk transfer produces a VfM superiority of $56.7 million in favour of the P3 (Infrastructure Ontario 2007b, 11).

Risk, in the context of a capital project, is held to be a situation of potential loss of investment resulting from operating in an uncertain business environment (Grimsey and Lewis 2004, 148–52). P3 justification rests on the normative claim that optimal risk transfer will produce the best VfM, and that the P3 model is uniquely able to achieve this. The most common risks attributed to P3 projects include site (tenure, access, suitability), design and construction (delays, weather, cost overruns), operation and maintenance (cost overruns), and financial risks (interest rates, inflation). What the P3 model attempts to do, from a public policy perspective, is transfer to the private partner as many of these risks as would be feasible, minimizing the exposure of the public partner and creating a built-in incentive for the private partner to generate project efficiencies and lower overall costs. For instance, it is common for P3 contracts to stipulate that payments to the private partner will begin only once the project is operational, and continued payment is based on meeting performance criteria (Hodge and Greve 2005, 52). However, optimal risk transfer with P3s occurs not when all risks are transferred to the private partner but when taken up by "whoever is best able to manage it," and in so doing VfM is achieved (Freedland 1998, 306). Offloading all risks to the private partner is thus neither desirable nor an appropriate justification for using a P3.

Freedland (1998, 307) argues that, at heart, risk-transfer arguments contain the inherent assumption that "a commercial bearing or insurance of public burdens is a beneficial thing in and of itself." The reasoning here is highly circular: P3 projects are justified (rhetorically and mathematically) exclusively through the normative logic of the P3 model itself, ignoring the option of transferring risk through traditional contracts (Ontario Auditor General 2008; Quebec Auditor General 2009). This level of self-referentiality fits squarely within the "rolling-with" variant of normalized neoliberalism described in the previous chapter.

An emphasis on risk transfer also relies upon the belief that failure, mis-estimation, and suboptimal performance are commonplace occurrences with public infrastructure and service provision, even when these beliefs may be completely unsubstantiated. For example, P3s are now used for most large public infrastructure projects in Ontario but, as confirmed by the former president and CEO of Infrastructure Ontario, there has yet to be any systematic analysis of the track record of risk and performance associated with traditional public procurement in that province (Ontario Standing Committee on Government Agencies 2008, 1130). Left unchecked, the underlying normative assumption that public procurement is inherently riskier incentivizes P3 use as a way of protecting against purportedly common risks – despite it being far from certain which (if any) particular risks bedevil public infrastructure projects. Assuming that public management is less efficient and effective also provides the rationale needed to blame the public sector should P3s perform worse than expected, justifying the appropriation of project-development techniques from the private sector and increasing public sector dependence upon market actors for their P3 knowledge and expertise.

Stripped of all rhetoric and self-promoting jargon, risk transfer through a P3 amounts to three things: privileging certain risks, ignoring others, and creating new risks along the way. The risks controlled (transferred) through a P3 are those that private partners can profit from or, in other words, those that the state can marketize and monetize by turning public goods and services into exchangeable commodities through competitive bidding and for-profit delivery. At the same time, risk assignment is based on the probability of particular outcomes, and thus it ignores future possibilities that cannot be stated statistically (Froud 2003, 570). Uncertain costs (unknown or unacknowledged risks) are not transferred and always remain with the state (581). The rigidness of the P3 contract precludes any subsequent transfer of uncompensated risks onto the shoulders of the private partner once the project agreement is signed.

It follows, therefore, that the risks (and uncertainties) that are not incorporated into VfM assessments are those that would discourage the use of P3s. Project risks are narrowly equated with market-derived conceptions of the public interest, which do not take into consideration concerns such as the contradiction that exists between profit-making and commercial confidentiality on the one hand, and democratic oversight and local control on the other. Collective risks associated with service-quality deterioration or more-precarious working conditions are similarly excluded.

Along with the simultaneous privileging and suppression of particular risks is the creation of risk and uncertainty through P3 use. Multi-decade-long contracts lock public service decision-making into "a particular pattern of service provision whereby changes must be negotiated with the provider and paid for" (Froud 2003, 580). This lock-in may stifle innovation and flexibility since the health sector requires that infrastructure be able to meet and adapt to future service needs and changes in policy and technology.

Even considered on its own terms, justification for risk allocation is often opaque. For example, with the Fredericton-Moncton Highway Project P3, the auditor general of New Brunswick affirmed that the request for proposals issued by the province clearly allocated most project risks to the private partner (development, design and construction risks; operation and maintenance risks; demand risks; and finance risks), and noted that this would provide for a significant transfer of risk above and beyond traditional forms of project procurement (New Brunswick Auditor General 1999, 68). However, when the auditor general attempted to investigate the basis on which these risks were transferred and assigned to the project partners (in order to establish value for money), he was "unable to develop any substantive evidence supporting risk transfer decisions" (85). Certainly the mere presence of a private for-profit partner alone is not enough to ensure these risks were advantageously transferred.

Scrutinizing Infrastructure Ontario's (IO) methodology, Loxley (2012, 19) points to the equally nebulous nature of risk transfer in Ontario:

The risk analysis of IO is based on a report from a private consultant (Infrastructure Ontario, 2007) which comes up with a risk transfer matrix showing that the province would retain risk equal to 43.6% of base construction costs under a traditional model and only 16.7% of base construction costs under a Build-Finance model. These, it argues would vary from project to project and it appears that the projects mentioned assume greater risk transfer than the average suggested by the consultants (over 3:1 versus the 2.6:1 implied in the model). The problem with the consultants' report is that there is no source, reference or justification given for any one of its numbers. None of the individual projects does any better as absolutely no support is presented, except the consultants' report, for the risk transfer figures given. If these crucial risk transfer numbers have any foundation empirically, it is not clear what it is or where it comes from.

Furthermore, in their study of P3s from the United Kingdom, Ireland, the Netherlands, Australia, and Denmark, Vining and Boardman (2008, 14) find that risk transfer as a central justification for P3s is inadequate as a P3 does not actually reduce risk, it merely reassigns it. As they suggest, given that governments can spread risks over a larger number of projects, it does not always follow that simply transferring all risks to the private partner leads to enhanced VfM (14). Not taking advantage of the potential for cost savings through risk pooling (i.e., publicly financing a large number of projects) can amount to a huge loss for the citizen and taxpayer. In his study of Alberta P3 schools, Hugh Mackenzie (2007, iv) found that "for every two schools financed using the P3 model, an additional school could be built if they were all financed using conventional public sector financing."

A final consideration, and perhaps the most damning for the risk-transfer argument, is that in order for the public partner to offload some or all of these risks, compensation for the acceptance of risk must be offered. This compensation translates into the anticipated profit margin of the private partner. Unless the private partner is inexperienced with P3s, this risk will be reflected in the price of the bids submitted to a request for proposals, or, as Grimsey and Lewis (2004, 179) summarize succinctly, "In risk allocation, nothing is free." Prospective private partners build risk premiums into their bids as a form of "self-insurance" (179). Private partners are therefore compensated for accepting certain project risks whether they arise or not, and indeed this is a major source of profit-making with P3s. As mentioned in chapter 1, taking responsibility for project risks can be a very lucrative arrangement, and shareholders involved with privately financed P3s tend to expect real rates of return on investment of at least 15–25 per cent per year (Gaffney et al. 1999, 116; Hodge 2004, 162). Justifying the use of a P3 on the basis of

risk transfer alone is therefore untenable, since qualified private partners will either avoid bidding on contracts that offload too much risk,
or this risk will be monetized in the form of higher-cost bids in line
with the anticipated profit margin sought by investors (Cohn 2004, 8).
Thus the monetization of risk through the bidding process cancels out
risk transfer as "risk becomes just one component of the project's cost
structure and is therefore passed completely onto the state in the consortium's bid" (Rouillard 2006, 5).

In sum, under the auspices of "risk transfer," private partners
assume responsibility for hypothetical project risks such as cost overruns and delays in exchange for lucrative investment opportunities.
Risk transfer, however, is illusory, not only because it is fully paid for
by the public partner rather than simply "transferred" to the private
partner, but also because calculations of risk in P3 value for money
assessments use biased methodology. As reported by the Institute for
Public Policy Research in Britain, "None of [the PFI hospital projects
on which data exist] show significant value for money savings when
set against the Public Sector Comparator. In the case of most NHS hospital PFI schemes the small projected savings could easily disappear if
some assumptions relating to risk, or the discount rate, were altered"
(as quoted in Farnsworth 2006, 833).

Value for Money Methodology

In order to ascertain whether a P3 is likely to be more or less costly than
a traditional project, best practice dictates that a public sector comparator (PSC) be generated in order to determine VfM. The PSC provides
the mechanism through which a P3 can be compared to a traditional
form of project delivery. Financial and quantifiable non-financial benefits are compared in both cases, and the option with the lowest net
present cost is typically chosen. There are, however, many controversial aspects to the VfM process, beyond those already mentioned above
with respect to cost savings and risk transfer.

First, an amount (known as a "risk adjustment") is added to the PSC
to cover risks like construction overruns and operational difficulties,
under the presumption that with a P3 the private partner will be contractually obligated to cover these risks. Broadbent, Gill, and Laughlin
(2003, 427) report that for P3s in the United Kingdom, nearly 50 per cent
of the total risk adjustment (the amount added to the PSC) is related
to design and construction risk valuation. However, as previously

mentioned, the auditors general of Ontario (2008) and Quebec (2009) argue that there is no reason to assume that risks relating to construction and design (among other things) cannot be adequately managed through a traditional design-build contract. Incorporating the assumption that a PSC would not be able to transfer this risk into VfM methodology is therefore a highly questionable practice.

Second, on top of the amount added to the PSC to cover risk, a discount rate is applied, which can significantly affect VfM calculations. Discounting is used to compare the two forms of cash – money spent today versus payments that are spread over many decades – and is based on the private sector principle that money spent today costs more since it had the potential to earn interest if spent gradually (Gaffney et al. 1999). It is held that discounting is necessary for VfM determinations as the cost of conventional projects is typically born upfront during the initial stages (the design and construction phase), whereas a P3 spreads costs over the entire project (Broadbent, Gill, and Laughlin 2003, 428). Through the application of a discount rate, net present costs can be calculated for both the P3 and PSC, and the lowest cost is taken to represent best VfM.

Aside from the fact that private sector techniques used to maximize shareholder value may not be wholly appropriate for determining public policy, the most controversial aspect of this practice is the discount rate chosen. The rate is so sensitive that it can easily skew the VfM calculation in favour of the P3 (Shaffer 2006; Gaffney et al. 1999; Parks and Terhart 2009). The higher the discount rate applied, the more attractive the P3 will appear, since money spent today becomes more costly. A few examples from BC make this clear.

When calculating VfM for the Diamond Centre hospital P3 in Vancouver, Partnerships BC used a discount rate of 7.12 per cent. To illustrate its sensitivity, Parks and Terhart (2009, 9) calculate that if a 4.12 per cent discount rate had been applied, the P3 would have represented a net present-value cost of $15.2 million over and above that of the PSC. However, if a 9.12 per cent discount rate had been applied, the P3 would appear to produce a net present-value savings of $29.6 million. With no discounting applied to the VfM assessment, the difference in nominal dollars is $114 million in favour of the PSC (10). Similarly, with the Sea-to-Sky highway P3, Partnerships BC applied a discount rate of 7.5 per cent; however at 5.0 per cent (the government's borrowing rate at the time) the P3 costs almost $220 million more than the PSC (Shaffer 2006, 6). As Loxley (2012, 2010) indicates, even though there is no globally agreed upon discount rate, rates used to calculate VfM in Ontario and BC are well above the UK best practice rate of 3.5 per cent, often by 1–3 per cent respectively. This practice makes it appear as though a P3 offers better value, even in cases where cost savings fail to materialize. International evidence produces similar results (e.g., Hodge and Duffield 2010).

The VfM appraisal process is also problematic because discounting is applied on top of the additional risk valuation added to the PSC. Gaffney et al. (1999) argue that in effect this double counts the cost of risk to the disadvantage of the PSC. Furthermore, returning to a previously discussed issue, P3 contracts provide market-based protections against *some* risks but they also ignore uncertain future scenarios and create new risks of their own. As Lyons (1996) reminds us, all contracts are inevitably incomplete and cannot possibly insure against every contingency in the future. However, "equivalent treatment of (existing) and created [P3] risks would require that the exposure to new risk be quantified and added to the private sector's bid as a potential cost that would not be incurred under conventional procurement and operation" (Froud 2003, 580). This practice is not followed with current VfM analyses, a methodological omission that clearly favours the P3 option.

P3 Hospitals

In addition to generic pitfalls associated with the P3 model are three unique concerns specific to P3 hospitals: they stifle innovation, create an internal bifurcation of authority, and unduly burden efforts of the third sector and resources of the local community.

The first concern is the mismatch between the fixed, contract-based mode of physical infrastructure planning and the long-run need for flexibility. Design innovation with hospitals relates specifically to the physical adaptability of the building, as it must meet today's needs whilst also accommodating future economic and social requirements as well as medical advances (Barlow and Köberle-Gaiser 2008). In 2001 the UK Department of Health (2001) reiterated the importance of health infrastructure-design innovation (conceptualized as adaptability) as a way of improving care at the same time as the PFI model had begun to proliferate within that sector. Several years later, case study evidence of PFI hospitals in the UK compiled by Barlow and Köberle-Gaiser (1392) led to the finding that "the PFI model is unable to promote the level of innovation in the design of hospital built assets needed to optimize their lifetime clinical efficiency."

Though the challenge of adaptability may be equally present with traditional hospitals, the nature of P3 contracts creates additional hurdles, given the nature of its project agreement arrangements: the length of the contract is both too long and too short to generate innovative solutions from a risk-based perspective. A critique applicable to all P3s, but particularly appropriate in the case of hospital projects, is the long-term, inflexible nature of the market-based contracts. This locks policy, design, and service planning in for several decades, whereas innovations in technology, public policy, and other related fields can have much shorter life cycles – making project agreements far too long within the health sector.

On the other hand, P3 contracts are also too short to truly transfer many important risks to the private partner. With average P3 hospital contract lengths of roughly thirty years, the P3 model can transfer some immediate risks associated with construction and maintenance, but the private consortia need only consider the medium-run design of a hospital, not the long-term and uncertain risks. Functional obsolescence, changing policies, and unidentified future health care needs fall onto the shoulders of the public sector, which holds ultimate responsibility for hospitals in perpetuity (Pollock, Shaoul, and Vickers 2002). Further, Leiringer (2006) finds that as a way of minimizing the costs associated with construction risk, P3 private partners have an incentive to use tried and true design and construction techniques, not the most forward-thinking and innovative ones. Thus design is conducted by profit-oriented risk-averse partners with little motivating them to plan for uncertain changes that would likely occur outside the parameters of the project agreement.

Hospital design from the perspective of private architectural and construction firms also represents a repository of knowledge and expertise, raising a related irony: rather than improving efficiency and fostering innovation, the competitive nature of P3 tendering discourages the very features it is purported to engender. When expertise in long-run infrastructure planning and design was held mainly in-house, efficiencies and innovations were generated through retained knowledge within the public sector. Privatizing this knowledge and subjecting it to (albeit limited) market competition individualizes hospitals from a design perspective, eliminating inter-project learning. Intra-project learning is also stifled as health-service planning becomes disintegrated from the design and operation of physical infrastructure. Since hospital project agreements in Canada do not cover clinical services, there is little incentive for the private partner to plan and design for the improvement of clinical care (Barlow and Köberle-Gaiser 2008).

Another problem specific to P3 hospitals is the contradiction between the privatized mode of support service-delivery and the need for clinical and non-clinical service integration within global hospital planning. Sometimes referred to as an "internal bifurcation of authority" (Shrybman 2007; Mehra 2005), this feature of P3 hospitals is produced when authority and oversight over hospital services is no longer held exclusively by public health authorities but shared with P3 private partners.

Problems associated with an internal bifurcation of authority include disintegrated planning procedures, and hindrances placed upon communication and collaboration within the hospital. The duplication of administrative layers and authority structures can also create problems related to uncertainty and inflexibility should labour disputes arise. This feature introduces private for-profit decision-making into the heart of medicare in Canada: hospital management and health-service planning. Not only is decision-making profit oriented but hospital boards (Ontario) and regional health authorities (BC) working with P3 operators are no longer in charge of monitoring support service contractors. With the P3 model, subcontracted service-providers become the responsibility of the private partner, making P3 support-service privatization distinct from contracting-out within traditional hospitals. Shrybman feels that the private financing and management of support services could facilitate the flourishing of two-tier health care, given that P3 hospitals allow private investors to "integrate, within the public hospital setting, a parallel and privately funded health services regime" (2007, 198).

With multi-decade project agreements, the higher costs associated with P3s are locked in over the long run, which can put pressure on managers of public health systems to make cuts in other areas in order to keep up with P3 payments. In the case of the Brampton Civic Hospital P3 (discussed in chapter 6), the province has assumed responsibility for the capital costs but not for the service contract, which falls onto the hospital board, as do the tough decisions and trade-offs that must be made in times of fiscal austerity. Given that severing the service component from the overall project agreement is subject to formalized contract-dispute procedures, it would be prohibitively expensive for a local public authority to contemplate this scenario – even in the case of poor performance.

Through a series of freedom-of-information requests in 2011, it has been revealed that NHS trusts in the UK are now locked into long-term PFI deals where they are "forced to pay 'hyper-inflated' charges for basic services" such as "£242 to put a padlock on a garden gate at a trust in North Staffordshire, £466 to replace a light fitting and £75 for an air freshener in Cumbria and £15,000 to 'install a laundry door following feasibility study' at a trust in Salisbury" (Hope 2012). Being locked into more-costly, long-running PFI deals also led to the June 2012 bankruptcy of South London Healthcare NHS Trust, and soon after it was revealed that an additional twenty-two NHS trusts faced "unsustainable" financial conditions as a result of expensive PFI hospitals (Alleyne 2012).

Serious financial problems of this sort have yet to surface in Canada, although in light of performance agreements that prohibit regional health authorities from running deficits, P3 payments will take priority over other service needs in Canada as well. In BC, for example, the provincial government had historically provided year-end bailouts of regional health authorities (RHAs) that were in danger of running a deficit. As of 2009, BC health minister Kevin Falcon had announced that these top-ups would no longer take place, forcing RHAs to cut hundreds of millions of dollars, achieved through service caps and cuts, slashed jobs, and higher user fees where applicable ("BC Health Authorities" 2009). School boards face similar spending constraints in the province, and in 2012 the provincial government fired the Cowichan Valley District 79 school board for not balancing the budget (Nuttall 2012). There is little reason to believe that provincial officials will not strongly enforce the balance budget imperative imposed on RHAs as well.

Lock-in is often viewed favourably by P3 proponents, cast as a mechanism of protection for the public, given that project agreements include performance-based payment schemes. With private partners subject to penalties and deductions, it is argued, the public is insulated from unnecessary cost and risk. In practice, P3 agreements are not always as robust as they appear. As discussed in chapter 5, with the Diamond Centre P3 in BC, despite claims to the contrary, payment deductions cannot be imposed, and the public partner cannot compel the private operator to seek out new subcontractors – even when a problem relates to an issue as serious as hospital infection control. Further, also discussed in chapter 5, often public partners prefer to resolve disputes through negotiation and compromise rather than imposing financial penalties on private partners.

The third concern specific to P3 hospitals in Canada is the additional burden that this model places on third-sector and municipal or community-based efforts and resources. Common to BC and Ontario is the stipulation that a portion of the infrastructure and equipment costs of all new hospitals (whether P3 or not) be paid through the contributions of local communities, known as the "local share." In Ontario the local share is the responsibility of public hospital corporations and the charitable organizations that participate in funding drives; in BC this is the responsibility of regional health authorities, regional hospital districts, hospital foundations, and auxiliaries.[1] Historically the local share has varied quite significantly in Ontario, oscillating from between zero and half of the cost associated with hospital equipment and furnishings (Ontario Standing Committee on Public Accounts 2009). In BC the local share component has been more stable and is often upwards of 40 per cent (Bish and Clemens 2008, 73).

Since the local share is a proportion of total costs rather than a fixed or risk-adjusted amount, as hospital costs grow, so too does the burden placed upon third-sector and community contributions. In the case of the Brampton Civic Hospital P3 (examined in chapter 6), additional costs became so great that the William Osler Health Centre (WOHC, the public hospital corporation) was unable to generate the local share of construction and equipment procurement and installation (Ontario Auditor General 2008, 118). The Ministry of Health was then forced to grant WOHC credits for the difference between what the public design-build costs would have been and the P3 bid, amounting to $164 million (118). The ministry has since revised its policy for local share contributions and this now stands at 10 per cent of the construction costs and 100 per cent of the equipment costs (124). In BC, the Fraser Valley Regional Hospital District contributed $72.3 million to the $355 million Abbotsford P3 (FVRD n.d.), or roughly 20 per cent of the capital cost.[2] Total capital costs associated with this P3 escalated by over 50 per cent between 2001 and 2008 and thus so too did the local share (see chapter 5 for more detail on cost creep).

---

1 Hospital foundations and auxiliaries are registered charities run by volunteers that finance equipment used in hospitals. Hospital foundations also help fund some clinical costs and research institutes, manage donation and investment income, and often run health and wellness campaigns.

2 The Fraser Valley Regional Hospital District falls under the purview of the Fraser Valley Regional District. Regional Districts in BC are not separate levels of government but instead are "federations of the municipalities and electoral areas that exist within their boundaries" (BC Ministry of Community Services 2005, 9). Their major revenue sources are property value taxes, parcel taxes, and fees and charges (8).

The relationship between P3s and the charitable/not-for-profit agents that contribute to the local share component of these hospitals differs slightly from the one more typically identified in the literature on the third sector and neoliberal restructuring. For example, in Evans and Shields (1998, 2000) on Canada, and Van Gramberg and Bassett (2005) on Australia, we read of the ways in which public sector rollback creates a greater reliance upon, and commercialization of, the third sector. In the Canadian health care sector the situation is somewhat different, given the relative insulation of medicare from neoliberal rollback, at least in comparison with other areas of welfare state policy. Medically necessary services remain publicly funded and provided, and smaller hospital projects are rarely delivered using private financing; similarly, hospital foundations, charities, and auxiliaries have retained their longstanding (pre-neoliberal) commitment to providing hospital equipment and funding certain other capital costs. Thus, with respect to the third sector and P3s, the more relevant changes taking place within Canada's public health sector are those that are occurring *within* the private sector (for-profit and not-for-profit) rather than between the public and third sectors. As for-profit entities begin to play a larger role in public health care, the role of not-for profit entities becomes subordinated in decision-making and influence. At the same time, private financing and service delivery can mean greater project costs, and thus greater fundraising pressures, placed on third-sector contributors.

Given the many problems associated with the use of P3s – misleading claims of risk transfer, accounting techniques used to make partnerships appear less costly, high transaction costs and ignored social costs, and systematic bias in the evaluation methodology – the obvious question becomes: why the continued proliferation of P3s? The answer offered here is that P3s are (and can only be) justified, whether overtly or implicitly, through an appeal to neoliberal ideals that favour dispossession and marketization and attempt to normalize this inherently normative policy. Even in cases where P3s may come in on time and on budget this cannot significantly offset the other transaction costs involved, the introduction of future policy inflexibility, and loss of full public control over vital infrastructure and services. In addition to these longstanding concerns, more recent problems have also emerged as a result of the 2008 global financial crisis.

Public-Private Partnerships and the 2008 Global Financial Crisis

Despite growing enthusiasm for P3s since the early 2000s, fortunes began to turn for this form of privatization with the onset of the recent global financial crisis. Most P3s are heavily reliant upon international bond markets for their financing, and the credit crunch that occurred in the wake of the crisis created a huge barrier to private financing. The year 2008 proved to be the worst year on record for P3s worldwide, with far fewer coming to financial close than had been the trend in recent years. Government support was soon tailored to rescuing P3s, and by 2010 their use began to rebound, thanks in part to financial market improvement but also to the support of steadfast state policy. This next section briefly chronicles these events: from collapsed and abandoned deals to their rescue by public policymakers. Government support took two principal forms: an encouragement of new projects, despite serious problems with the private finance portion of P3s; and the creation of P3 units and P3-targeted financing schemes to rescue projects and promote new P3s.

Collapsed and Abandoned P3 Deals

Private financing for P3s is typically split between debt and equity. An equity stake involves fundamental ownership rights over the P3's private partner (a firm, consortium, or special project vehicle), entitling asset holders to revenue after costs are met and debt obligations paid (Hellowell and Vicchi 2012, 7). Debt holders are not granted property rights over the P3 but are guaranteed interest and capital repayment and are given a higher priority over cash flows (purportedly to incentivize good project management by equity holders) (ibid). Debt during the construction phase of a project is often secured through private commercial banks, with bond financing used for the operational phase. Stakeholder investors (equity holders) are typically engineering, procurement, construction, operations, and maintenance firms; project investors (debt holders) are usually pension funds, sovereign wealth funds, infrastructure funds, and banks (public investment banks and private commercial banks) (Waterston 2012). The split between debt and equity (or "gearing ratio") with privately financed P3s tends towards 90 per cent debt and 10 per cent equity. However, the total capital cost of a P3 project may not be drawn entirely from private finance. It has been noted that a distinctive feature of the "Canadian model" is the use of large amounts of public money upfront (Siemiatycki 2012). With the $2.1 billion Canada Line in Vancouver, for example, only one third of the capital costs were covered privately.

The use of private debt and equity financing to deliver public infrastructure has long been criticized as a key factor in the comparatively higher costs of P3s (e.g., Hellowell and Pollock 2007; Loxley 1999a; 1999b; 2010). This results from the interest rate differential that typically exists between private sector and public sector borrowers. Governments in Canada generally receive better credit ratings, and thus pay lower interest rates, than the private sector, since they uniquely hold the power of general taxation to guarantee that all debts will be honoured. This long-standing issue of higher-priced P3 projects was made even worse by the recent global financial crisis, as costs associated with the private finance portion of newly initiated partnerships were ratcheted up significantly.

Prior to 2007, government borrowers in Canada were able to secure interest rates that were, on average, 2 per cent lower than those charged to private borrowers, but between 2007 and 2009 this increased to an average of 3 or 4 per cent – making P3s nearly 70 per cent more expensive than publicly funded infrastructure when measured in present value terms (Mackenzie 2009, 2). Globally, transaction costs also increased as the time-frame for negotiations was lengthened due to financial market instability (Drapak 2009). Several years on, private finance costs remain high, even in the face of historically low prime rates throughout the 2009–10 global recession. Given that a P3 private partner is often structured as a special purpose vehicle, lenders have recourse only to the assets created through the P3, not all assets of the borrowers. P3 rates thus far exceed government bond rates and even many corporate bond rates. In the United Kingdom, as of late 2013, private financing came in at roughly 7–8 per cent, whereas the yield on a twenty-year UK Gilt was just over 4 per cent, pushing capital costs up by 3–4 per cent (Hellowell 2013). Throughout the global financial crisis in particular, the combination of higher financing and transaction costs significantly affected P3 value for money.

Operating alongside this widening public/private interest-rate spread were changes in financial market dynamics. Prior to 2007, P3s were often financed through project bonds, as opposed to bank loans. Money for a project would be raised when individual and institutional investors purchased these assets through monoline bond markets. In exchange for a fee, monoline insurers would take on the risk that returns on the bond would be lower than what the lender expected. Through this guarantee (or wrap) the asset was usually assigned a credit rating equal to that of the monoline insurers themselves (typically AAA), resulting in much lower interest rates than otherwise available through bank loans (for more on monoline, see Tett 2007). The high credit rating allowed institutional investors with particular creditworthiness requirements, such as pension funds, to purchase these bonds.

Throughout the early to mid-2000s, monoline companies began insuring mortgage-backed securities and wrapping other high-risk assets later implicated in the subprime debt crisis, leading to a loss of investment grade ratings and even to bankruptcies and nationalization. Whereas in late 2007 there were six monoline insurers that carried a triple A credit rating – Ambac Assurance Corporation, CIFG Guaranty, Financial Guaranty Insurance Company (FGIC), Financial Security Assurance (FSA), MBIA Insurance Corporation, and XL Capital Assurance – within a few short years, each had lost its investment grade status or worse. XL Capital Assurance was downgraded far below investment grade in mid-2008, CIFG was at "junk" status in 2008, FSA and MBIA were both rated as speculative grade (below A) in 2009, Ambac filed for bankruptcy protection in 2010, and FGIC was bankrupt and temporarily nationalized in 2012.

When the option to secure monoline-wrapped bonds disappeared, there was a near-overnight elimination of the main source of private financing used in P3 deals. The upheaval associated with higher cost and more difficult to secure private financing led to a series of delays, renegotiations, and collapsed deals in 2008/9.

In Canada the effects of the financial crisis began to show in mid-2008, and most projects that reached financial close at this time were smaller in scope and required only short-term financing (CCPPP 2009, 1). Several high-profile and high-cost deals were affected. With the Port Mann Bridge P3, one of the private partners (Macquarie Infrastructure Group) was unable to come up with the requisite $700 million, and as a result the province of British Columbia was forced to renegotiate the agreement in order to keep the project going (Hunter 2009). This renegotiation occurred just weeks before construction was scheduled to begin. With the Fort St John Hospital P3 project, also in BC, financial market instability meant that a new private partner was needed to bail out the original private-equity provider contracted to finance the $268 million hospital (Mackenzie 2009, 11). Although the BC provincial government remained committed to actively pursuing P3 projects throughout the crisis, stimulus fund spending targeted speedier traditional infrastructure projects, and decision-makers suspended the requirement that P3s be first considered for all large infrastructure projects (10). The requirement that P3s must be first considered for all large infrastructure projects has since been reimposed.

Other pro-P3 provinces faced similar problems. In Ontario, for example, the Niagara Health Systems P3 project, originally scheduled to begin construction in spring 2009, was delayed for several months when the private financing portion fell through (Mackenzie 2009, 12).

A new private financing partner then stepped in. Rather than abandon P3 policy altogether, the province temporarily moved away from partnerships arrangements that relied on private financing.

International comparisons produce similar results. In the United Kingdom, 2008 and 2009 were the lowest-volume years on record since 1998 when the PFI heyday began. During the height of the financial crisis, the average number of P3 projects to reach financial close had been cut in half, with only thirty-four and thirty-five projects closing, in 2008 and 2009 respectively (Timmins 2010). For this reason, in 2009 the United Kingdom launched its PFI Lending Initiative to finance projects that would have otherwise been terminated due to a shortfall in private sector lending (CCPPP 2009, 6).

Worldwide the volume of P3 deals was stagnant in 2008, and by mid-2009 25 per cent of all P3 deals had been cancelled (Drapak 2009). Higher-cost private financing also meant that interest rate spreads in newly industrialized and developing countries (where global P3 growth had previously been most prominent just prior to the crisis) increased to levels not seen since the Asian Financial Crisis in 1997 (Berger et al. 2009, 5). Operational P3s in these emerging market countries faced problems with refinancing similar to those experienced in Canada. However, unlike in Canada, the global economic downturn in 2009 greatly affected newly proposed P3s, since revenue for projects in developing countries tends to rely on direct user fees (e.g., tolls). The recession thus cut into the revenue streams relied upon by P3 investors, narrowing the range of prospective bidders. Exchange rate fluctuations also caused many developing countries' projects to be cancelled (7). A study conducted by the World Bank's Public-Private Infrastructure Advisory Facility between 2008 and 2009 reported that roughly one-third of the developing countries polled experienced delays with P3 projects, with South Asia and transitional economies in Europe and Central Asia accounting for the majority (13). All of this has led industry experts to conclude that "none would suggest that the PPP market is likely to return to the ideal conditions in previous years" (CCPPP 2009, 1). The historical low point in the global P3 market (late 1990s / early 2000s) may be the new "normal" in the volume of annual P3 deals (Leigland and Russell 2009, 4).

Despite the problems identified above, it is equally true that Canadian P3 markets enjoyed relative stability throughout the global financial crisis given that this country has a comparatively well-developed infrastructure bond market to finance P3 deals (see Dunsky and Stougiannos 2013;

Hoser, Gilbert, and Adams 2012; "Infrastructure Bonds" 2012; Project Finance 2011). These are unwrapped bonds that do not now, nor prior to the global financial crisis, rely on monoline insurers. Investment-grade ratings are instead secured through investment-grade contractors, high-rated government partners, bonding support for contractors and subcontractors, and with major commercial banks as underwriters. Examples of P3 bond-financed projects in Canada include Montreal super-hospitals McGill University Health Centre (MUHC) and the Centre hospitalier universitaire de Montréal (CHUM), the relocation and consolidation of RCMP E Division Headquarters in metro Vancouver, and the Montreal-Laval Highway 25 toll bridge.

A more problematic feature of Canadian P3 private financing schemes is a reliance upon "mini-perm" finance structures. Mini-perm financing refers to when the tenor of a project's senior debt is much shorter than the duration of the P3 project agreement (Hellowell and Vicchi 2012). Refinancing will typically be required within the first five to seven years of a thirty-year (or greater) contract. Under the assumption that projects could be refinanced periodically at projected rates, many existing P3s have secured financing for a shorter term than the life of the project. Mackenzie (2009) suggests that the rationale underpinning privately financed P3s therefore had a built-in expectation that the credit-fuelled bubble would continue indefinitely. There was little prudence demonstrated, despite P3 proponents often justifying partnerships on the basis of fiscal austerity, and promoters did not factor in the possibility of a looming financial crisis. Fiscal recklessness such as this led Scotland's finance minister John Swinney to label the use of private financing associated with P3s "one of the worst excesses of the age of financial irresponsibility" (Fraser 2009). The global financial crisis and its immediate aftermath also led several Canadian policymakers to publicly question their use. For instance, Quebec health minister Yves Bolduc stated in 2009 that "P3s were not a religion" for his party (CUPE 2009). The Treasury Board president, minister of transport, and minister of municipal affairs also cast doubt on the future of P3s in that province, and several proposed P3s were scrapped in favour of public procurement (CUPE 2009).

P3 Rescue: Government Promotion and Support

Despite serious problems with P3 markets in 2008–9, several Canadian provinces continued to initiate new P3s throughout the crisis. BC and

Ontario in particular remained committed, announcing new infrastructure projects in areas relating to health care, transportation, incarceration, water treatment, and other important sectors throughout the crisis and recession (see Partnerships BC, n.d.; Infrastructure Ontario, n.d.).

One way in which this was accomplished in BC was through the alteration of certain private-financing accounting rules. Given the sudden increase in private sector borrowing costs relative to government borrowing, in 2009 Partnerships BC began to use a "wide equity" financing model, temporarily suspending the requirement that a private partner provide both equity and bank financing (Partnerships BC 2009). Thus for the Fort St John Hospital P3 the government took on the loan risk, and the private partner (ISL Health) was allowed to increase its equity share (from 10 per cent to 14 per cent) (Reynolds 2012). This significantly reduced the burden of financial-risk transfer for the private partner as the Northern Health Authority came to assume most of the cost of construction. Although the wide-equity model did save taxpayers from some of the additional costs associated with private financing during the crisis, a portion of the project's financing still came from more expensive private debt. Coupled with the lack of significant risk transfer, this raises the obvious question of why a P3 arrangement was needed at all for this project.

Support for individual projects was also accompanied by longer-term initiatives such as the creation of P3 units – specialized government agencies charged with promoting and assisting with P3 development (helping with project financing and offering technical and legal guidance). At the federal level in Canada, PPP Canada Inc. now takes up this task. Created in late 2007 as a federal Crown corporation, PPP Canada promotes, assesses and evaluates, and provides expertise and assistance with the development of partnerships across the country (and at the municipal level in particular). Once the P3 market deteriorated sharply in 2008, PPP Canada also engaged in "extensive discussions" in 2008/9 with the provinces/territories, private sector stakeholders, and other federal organizations to gauge the nature and extent of public sector support needed to ensure that new projects were started, and that recently initiated projects reached financial close. Through these efforts PPP Canada determined that its priority would be to help ease the "significant roadblock" to P3 projects posed by the financial crisis (PPP Canada 2009). In furtherance of its mandate to "develop the Canadian market for public-private partnerships," it received funding commitments from the federal government of $2.8 billion per annum for 2011–13. PPP Canada also teamed up with Export Development Canada to provide surety, bonding support, and co-lending to enable troubled P3 projects to proceed. Budget 2013 renewed these funding commitments once more, this time by $1.25 billion (Government of Canada 2013, chapter 3.3, "The New Building Canada Plan"). In contrast, fiscal austerity made a comeback at the federal level in Budget 2012, which introduced cuts totalling $5.2 billion (Government of Canada 2012).

Other countries have enacted similar forms of political support for P3s. In the United Kingdom, the Treasury created its PFI Lending Initiative in 2009 in order to provide financing for projects that would have otherwise been terminated as the result of a shortfall in private sector lending (CCPPP 2009, 6). In December 2009 the Chancellor of the Exchequer also announced in a pre-budget report the creation of Infrastructure UK (IUK) which "would take on the role to advise the Government on strategic long-term infrastructure planning, prioritization, financing and delivery across sectors from energy and waste, to water, telecommunications and transport" (Farquharson and Encinas 2010, 7). This brought together the Treasury's P3 policymakers, the country's P3 unit (Partnerships UK), and the new lending initiative as a way of integrating P3 policy into long-run infrastructure planning. France incorporated financial support for P3 initiatives into its 2008 stimulus plan (8). In contrast, the 2009 Canadian stimulus package suspended the 2007 requirement that P3s be considered first for large infrastructure projects (CLC 2009, 3–4), but this P3 screen was reimposed in 2011.

The active promotion of P3s during and after the 2008 crisis does more than merely allow P3 policy to move forward; it also encouraged a re-establishment of neoliberal rule through dispossession and marketization (a topic returned to in the concluding chapter). Further, the embracing of private finance to fund public services and infrastructure encourages risky practices such as off-balance-sheet accounting and the transformation of public goods into private assets to be traded and sold within opaque and volatile secondary financial markets (as securities or derivatives), with risks ultimately backed by the taxpayer. The commercial confidentiality that accompanies all P3 agreements also encourages low levels of corporate accountability and they allow for profit-seeking behaviour using market refinancing and equity sales – practices that are largely beyond public control once a project agreement is in place (see Reynolds 2011; Sandborn 2008; Whitfield 2009).

Concluding Remarks

P3s are a form of privatization that holds unique characteristics, distinguishing partnerships from full-scale asset divestiture and from more limited forms of contracting-out. An important part of the P3 process is the normalization of normative discourse and market-derived techniques, reframing notions of public infrastructure and service provision. Through a market-based conceptualization of risk, risk transfer, value for money, and cost savings, the traditional fully public option is evaluated against the P3 model in a way that is conceptually and methodologically biased in favour of privatization. The traditional method is no longer considered on its own terms and measured against its own strengths; nor is the P3 option subject to the values and outcomes of public procurement and collective decision-making. Risks created by P3s are not considered in value for money assessments, and neither are the risks that market-based transactions are unable to address. Self-referentiality of this sort brings specific problems to the health care sector: stifling innovation, locking-in particular policies when flexibility is far more desirable, draining resources through the introduction of profit, disintegrating service provision and hospital management, and subjecting public services and infrastructure to financial market volatility.

Chapter 3

Normalizing P3 Procurement

This chapter discusses the phases of P3 development that have shaped the Canadian landscape and explains how one phase has shifted into the next. Having originally emerged in the 1990s era of fiscal austerity, P3s were initially used in jurisdictions and sectors scattered across the country, justified mainly through an appeal to cost savings and off-book financing. In the past decade, P3 use has expanded greatly and is now the dominant form of procurement for large-scale infrastructure projects developed in the BC and Ontario provincial health sector. This current phase is distinguished by the creation and sophistication of sector-wide P3 programs, a concept that will be explored with reference to the institutional and procedural similarities and differences that have emerged in Ontario and BC. The two major phases of P3 development in Canada can also be understood in terms of the relative degree to which this form of dispossession has been routinized, institutionalized, and depoliticized – the subject of chapter 4.

Sector-wide P3 programs do not stand on their own; rather they are nested within wider provincial P3-enabling fields. Enabling fields are the other major policy innovation contributing to the flourishing of Canadian P3 hospitals over the past decade. The concept of an enabling field encapsulates a number of regulatory, procedural, and legal-institutional changes. In contrast, full-scale privatization might require only one piece of enabling legislation (e.g., the privatization of Air Canada through Bill C-29 in 1988). The multifaceted nature of P3-enabling fields attests once more to the uniqueness of P3s when compared with other forms of privatization that exist in Canada. With P3s dispossession occurs *within* the realm of the state, and marketization involves not only an expansion of market rule but also the adoption of market-like rules by the public sector. Partnerships should thus not be conflated with full-scale privatization (where public obligations are severed and private owners come to fully control the asset or service), nor are they limited to the privatized execution of policy choices made within the public sector (as is the case with contracting-out). The entrenchment of P3 procurement is thus a contingent phenomenon – requiring the historical and contemporary occupation of certain sectors and services by the state – and is reliant upon the ascension of a particular ideology or governance paradigm: neoliberalism and its emphasis on New Public Management and neoclassical economics. Further, neoliberalism can be subdivided into various forms, and it is within the rollout phase that P3s and enabling fields take root.

The central elements of the P3-enabling fields set up by Canada's key P3 enthusiasts, the BC and Ontario Liberal governments, examined in this chapter are legislation and capital planning frameworks; supportive secondary reforms; and new forms of institutional support. The legislative and capital planning framework changes relevant here are BC's Capital Asset Management Framework and Ontario's Infrastructure Planning, Financing, and Procurement Framework; and BC's Health Sector Partnerships Agreement Act and Ontario's Alternative Financing and Procurement model. Supportive secondary reforms refer to the 2001 restructuring of BC's regional health authorities and the 2006 initiation of Local Health Integration Networks in Ontario. New institutional support for P3s in each province is now provided by specialized P3 units, named Partnerships BC and Infrastructure Ontario.

Phases of Canadian P3 Development

Infrastructure P3s have existed in Canada since the mid-1990s, although several divisions within the timeframe of their existence have been proposed. Two principal divisions relate to those that emphasize changes in the political rationale provided to justify P3 use, and those anchored on the public sector institutional changes that support P3 development. The differing accounts of various eras of P3 development in Canada can be usefully cobbled together to form a more complete picture.

John Loxley (2010, 40–1) suggests three phases of P3 development. First was the emergence of a highly politicized, ideologically driven era in the mid-1990s. P3s were adopted at this time as a way of reducing the size of the public sector in accordance with rollback neoliberalism (e.g., P3s initiated by the Harris Progressive Conservative government in Ontario). Second, in the late-1990s to early 2000s Loxley argues that the rationale shifted slightly, from one that was strongly or overtly ideological to one that relied upon the purported financial and economic superiority of P3s. Finally, since the mid-2000s, he suggests that we have seen a re-emergence of "a purely political rationale" (40), indicated by the application of a P3 screen to federal infrastructure spending and the aggressive promotion of partnerships at the provincial level in select jurisdictions (BC, Ontario, Alberta, and Quebec).

The industry publication *Infrastructure Investor* ("Canada: An Intelligence Report" 2010, 6) also identifies three phases, but with its slightly different interpretation of the second and third phases it has a more institutionally oriented approach overall. From this perspective, the first stage began in the 1990s when all three levels of government developed P3s as "a way to try to get some off-balance sheet financing" (quoting Cynthia Robertson, executive director of the Canadian Council for Public-Private Partnerships, 6). This was followed by a second phase that began in the early 2000s when provinces such as Ontario and BC began to promote P3s as a way of capturing cost savings and efficiency gains, and created P3 units as procurement agencies and centres of excellence. Finally, the third and current phase is demarcated by the federal government's 2009 creation of PPP Canada. It is suggested that in this current phase the federal government will "take a stronger leadership role in coordinating private investment in infrastructure" (6).

A third phase-related interpretation that is more clearly distinguished by institutional innovations within the public sector is represented by a Conference Board of Canada publication (Iacobacci 2010), which argues that there have been only two eras, divided according to the absence/presence of specialized government agencies devoted to P3 promotion. The second phase thus began with those projects "that reached financial close under the auspices of the P3 agencies (or offices) set up in the early 2000s" (1). Colverson (2012) suggests that government "maturity" is a very important factor in the development of P3 markets. To be discussed shortly, here it is argued that maturation in Canada's leading P3-promoting provinces has meant shifting from individual one-off projects to focusing on sector-wide P3 programs that target areas earmarked for infrastructure renewal, such as health care. P3 programs are also supported by the creation of P3-enabling fields that provide a province-wide shape to P3 development.

The various justifications and forms of institutional support for P3 development identified by Loxley (2010), *Infrastructure Investor*

("Canada: An Intelligence Report" 2010), and the Conference Board of Canada (Iacobacci 2010) correspond to wider changes in neoliberal policy experienced over the past two decades, with practices shifting between the overtly ideological (normative) and the technocratic/ pragmatic (normalized). The rollback, rollout, and rolling-with variants of neoliberalization identified by Peck and Tickell (2002) and Keil (2009) are relevant here. As a subset of neoliberal policy, privatization also takes many forms – ranging from full-scale asset divestiture to contracting-out to P3s – and so too do the normative and normalized forms of support for P3s across the neoliberal era.

Both how policymakers justify P3s (i.e., rhetorically and ideologically) and the mechanisms through which the state is restructured to accommodate and encourage this phenomenon (i.e., legally and institutionally) are equally important.[1] The concept of an enabling field and its normalization of P3 procurement addresses both. But first, before examining the items that form the BC and Ontario P3-enabling fields, it is important to situate this discussion within another major corresponding policy development: the shift from a project-focus to a program-focus in key sectors.

The Shift from Projects to Programs

In light of the poor track record of early (1990s) P3s in Canada,[2] P3 proliferation continues and has gained prominence in Ontario and BC under Liberal governments over the past decade (beginning in 2003 and 2001, respectively), through the shift from a project- to a program-based focus. Longevity of the P3 model in these jurisdictions has been accomplished not through any significant resolution of the larger problems and conflicts that are inherent to this procurement model, but instead by shifting from the development of one-off projects to instead creating P3 programs within suitable sectors (mainly health care and transportation). The need to consider project size, scope, and opportunity for innovation and risk transfer tends to restrict the types of

---

1 Note that the relevant literature on this subject remains relatively mute about any changes required on the part of the private partner: for capital, the arrangement merely has to be profitable and predictable, which are qualities dictated largely by how committed and enthusiastic governments are for partnerships.

2 For example, see Loxley (2010) on the Hamilton-Wentworth water and sewage system (Ontario), Evergreen Park School (New Brunswick), Confederation Bridge (federal), Charleswood Bridge (Manitoba), and Highway 407 (Ontario).

Table 1. P3 Project, Program, Enabling Field

P3 project	An individual piece of infrastructure and its support services, governed by a project agreement, with a legally circumscribed public partner and private partner
P3 program	The sum of all P3 projects in a particular sector and their implementation regime; influenced by individual projects and the wider P3-enabling field yet containing issues, elements, hurdles, and stakeholders unique to a given program
P3-enabling field	The constellation of legal and institutional arrangements that facilitate, encourage, and allow for P3 projects and programs; inherently transformative (influencing pre-existing structures and relationships) and continually adapting to new circumstances and challenges; largely responsible for ridding jurisdictions of the pre-existing bias towards traditional project procurement through routinizing, institutionalizing, and depoliticizing dispossession (RID; see chapter 5)

projects and conditions most suitable for P3s (see Murphy 2008); however, large greenfield capital projects within health and transportation sectors most often fit these criteria.[3] P3 programs have in turn helped to build up the high level of specialized knowledge, expertise, experience, and commitment needed to pursue dispossession within the public sector. The web of support offered to projects and programs, or the "P3-enabling field," is the mechanism through which this shift is initiated. These distinctions are summarized in table 1.

The terms "program" and "enabling field" used in the table differ from other interpretations of P3 implementation (e.g., Greenaway, Salter, and Hart 2004; Jooste, Levitt, and Scott 2010; Jooste and Scott 2012; Rachwalski and Ross 2010). For instance, when Rachwalski and Ross (2010) use the term "P3 program" they are referring to P3s in all sectors, but here it is used in a more narrow fashion, as in fact P3 development can differ greatly from one sector to another. Sectoral differences are related to a number of factors. Canadian provincial health sectors, for example, have their own implementation regimes (relating to capital procurement procedures, the authorities and stakeholders involved, the level of public engagement, and other legal considerations

---

3 In contrast, PPP Canada (2013) has warned that the P3 model in its current form may not be suitable for addressing the need for new and upgraded water and wastewater infrastructure in Canada, given that these are typically small brownfield projects with complex risks.

such as the 1984 Canada Health Act, which bans user fees) that are not accounted for when "program" refers to all P3s within a given jurisdiction. Similarly, Jooste and Scott (2012, 151) focus on how enabling fields help overcome government, market, and other related difficulties experienced by P3s, but for them the enabling field is composed of a "network of new 'enabling organizations' (public, private, nonprofit)." The enabling organizations that they are referring to are, for example, specialized P3 units, auditors general, private consultants, and advocacy organizations. These organizations are no doubt crucial to the maturation of P3 markets, but focusing only on organizations (essentially the "institutional support" category of the enabling field as presented in this chapter) ignores the legislation, capital planning frameworks, and supportive secondary reforms that are particularly important for P3 programs in Canada. Use of the word "field" is highly relevant as well: with the notable exception of supportive secondary reforms specific to particular sectors, the elements that comprise provincial P3-enabling fields inform decision-making across the bureaucracy and public sector.

P3-Enabling Fields

The three elements present in Ontario and BC P3-enabling fields, along with examples of their primary components, are summarized in table 2. Note that prior to the creation of enabling fields there had been no provincial infrastructure P3s developed in BC, and Ontario had but a few

Table 2. P3-Enabling Fields

	BC	Ontario
Enabling legislation and capital planning frameworks	Community Charter Act (2003)	Municipal Act (2006)
	Capital Asset Management Framework (CAMF) (2002)	Infrastructure Planning, Financing, and Procurement Framework (IPFP) (2004)
	The Health Sector Partnerships Agreement Act (Bill 94) (2003)	Alternative Financing and Procurement model (AFP) (2004)
Supportive secondary reforms	Regional health authority (RHA) restructuring (2001)	Local Health Integration Network (LHIN) creation (2006)
Institutional support	Partnerships BC (PBC) (2002)	Infrastructure Ontario (IO) (2005)

projects in sectors at the municipal and provincial level, and no hospital P3s were yet operational.

Enabling Legislation and Capital Planning Procedures

This category accounts for the nuts and bolts of the P3-enabling field: the legislative and policy changes that are necessary for developing P3 projects and programs. A range of items are included, from those that facilitate and regularize P3 development (AFP, Bill 94), to those that coerce public sector bureaucrats to contemplate and evaluate the P3 option (CAMF, IPFP), and those that simplify P3 adoption at the municipal level (Community Charter Act, Municipal Act).

BC's Community Charter Act

The basic tenets of municipal government in BC, as identified by Bish (1990, 9; taken from Smith, Ginnell, and Black 2010, 247) are that "municipalities operate under rules set out by the province, they are mandated by the provincial government to perform certain administrative activities, and any actions undertaken by these municipalities have to be authorized by provincial legislation." These powers are not constitutionally entrenched, given that municipalities are (to repeat the cliché) "creatures of the provinces." Municipal powers were, however, recently augmented through legislative changes introduced in 2004 by Premier Campbell when the Community Charter Act was enacted.[4]

Of the new powers introduced through the Community Charter, four are particularly relevant to the development of future P3s (see Charter 2003, chapter 26, part 3; Smith and Stewart 2005; Smith, Ginnell, and Black 2010):

1 Within the boundaries of the constitution, municipalities are now allowed to establish any service they consider necessary.
2 Without prior provincial government approval, municipalities can now enter into partnership agreements with private entities in water, sewage, transportation, and gas, electrical, or other energy supply system.

---

4 Vancouver is the one exception in the province, as its power, authority, and operations were set out in the 1953 Vancouver Charter, which governs only the City of Vancouver.

3 The counter-petition process initially established in the Local Government Act has been watered down by increasing the proportion of the local population needed to sign a petition before a new bylaw or large spending project can be subject to a referendum, and by making referenda binding only if they fail.

4 The Community Charter also opens up the possibility, though it does not guarantee, that municipalities will be granted new ways to raise revenue beyond their historical reliance on property taxes (e.g., allowing them to apply new forms of taxation like entertainment and hotel taxes, to establish road tolls, and to enact user fees on various services.

These changes were promoted as a way of improving local governance by giving municipalities more flexibility and autonomy than they previously had, increasing accountability and good governance, and generating efficiencies through decentralization (Community Charter 2003; Smith and Stewart 2005; Smith, Ginnell, and Black 2010; "Accountability Is Missing" 2003). So far these benefits have been more rhetorical than actual, as accountability has been eroded ("Accountability Is Missing" 2003), the provincial government can still "override any local government on any project it deems 'of significant provincial interest'" (Smith, Ginnell, and Black 2010, 249), and fears that decentralization is merely a euphemism for cost and responsibility shifting have been raised (Depner 2002). In many ways the promise of greater autonomy and better, more democratic forms of local governance has yet to materialize.[5] Instead what these regulatory reforms more clearly achieve is the promotion and simplification of the municipal P3 development process. Thus the Community Charter is a prime example of neoliberal re-regulation allowing for dispossession at the local level.

The time and paperwork ("red tape") previously associated with establishing municipal P3s has now been reduced, and the legal impediments and associated delays that may have previously discouraged P3

5 In 2012, the BC provincial government announced the creation of an Auditor General for Local Government (AGLG) in order "make sure British Columbians are getting the best value for their money" (BC Office of the Premier 2012). The idea of introducing a spending watchdog at the municipal level originated with the BC Chamber of Commerce, and when the AGLG position was announced, the president of the Union of BC Municipalities admitted that some communities were opposed to the idea (Bailey 2012). This new position could have a significant impact on municipalities' autonomy and local democracy in the future.

ventures at the local level have been eliminated. Less red tape translates into enhanced freedom to enter into P3 agreements, and P3s can be used to provide any new service within a municipality's legal and juris-dictional purview – making it far easier to turn new services into com-modities. The ability to hold city council accountable for unpopular P3s at an early stage in their development has also been curtailed through changes to the regulations surrounding counter-petition. In addition, by allowing municipalities to create new revenue sources by imposing user fees, the tax increases that would otherwise prove necessary to afford new P3s are not required, thus avoiding "concerns in the business com-munity," as Ted Nebbeling, minister of state for the Community Charter, put it (quoted in Palmer 2003, 18). The ability to more easily apply user fees to new services and infrastructure also makes P3 revenue both more lucrative and assured for the private investor. Finally, municipalities have now been given the ability to grant tax holidays to businesses, effectively shifting the burden of more costly P3 repayment onto residents.

Ontario's Municipal Act

Municipalities in Ontario are also governed mainly by provincial leg-islation. The 2001 Municipal Act (and later the 2006 Municipal Statute Law Amendment Act, both to be referred to simply as the "Municipal Act") was introduced in order to "provid[e] local governments with new broad powers and significant legislative freedoms," giving municipali-ties "more autonomy" (Ontario Ministry of Municipal Affairs and Hous-ing 2007). Enhanced natural person rights (greater decision-making authority and independence) and control over services promote P3s in Ontario municipalities, much like the Community Charter does in BC. Natural person powers allow municipalities to enter into agreements (and conduct other types of business) without needing to seek or be given prior provincial approval.

In particular, section 110 of the Municipal Act (2001) grants municipal-ities the ability to "enter into agreements for the provision of municipal capital facilities by any person" – where "any person" includes a private sector entity. Capital facilities covered here include sectors suitable for P3s: electrical facilities; municipal facilities for telecommunication, tran-sit, and transportation; waste management, water and sewer facilities; municipal housing facilities; and community centres, libraries, and cul-tural facilities. While user fees within the public health care system are prohibited by the 1984 Canada Health Act, in other areas the application of tolls and fees can be a great boon for P3 development, given that it often means greater revenue for investors.

The Community Charter Act and Municipal Act are therefore forms of enabling legislation in the sense that they help ease the development of P3s at the municipal level by simplifying and accelerating implementation (granting greater autonomy to local decision-makers) and by providing new revenue sources from which P3s can be financed (helping to lure investors). However, these pieces of legislation in no way compel municipalities to adopt P3s. More coercive features of provincial P3-enabling legislation are the new public infrastructure procurement policy frameworks (the CAMF and IPFP) that now guide decision-making in BC and Ontario.

BC's Capital Asset Management Framework

In May 2002, the Capital Asset Management Framework (CAMF) was introduced to serve as new "rules of the road" for public infrastructure building in BC, governed by five best-practice principles: sound fiscal management, strong accountability, value for money, protection of the public interest, and competition and transparency (BC Ministry of Finance 2002, 1–2). The CAMF applies province-wide, and thus all ministries, public sector agencies, and other public organizations must now comply with these rules when seeking approval and funding for infrastructure projects.

When it was introduced, the Ministry of Finance made an effort to present the CAMF as being pragmatic, claiming that it "does not predetermine that every project will be a public-private partnership" (BC Ministry of Finance 2002, 1). Further, the Value for Money CAMF document states, "The framework does not assume that any one sector is inherently more efficient in building and operating public assets. Instead, it emphasizes that capital decisions will be based on a practical, project-specific assessment of a full range of options" (BC Ministry of Finance n.d., 5). Yet pragmatism is merely a mask for the dispossession-promoting evaluation that makes up the bulk of CAMF procedures. In order to fulfil lofty principles like achieving the best value for taxpayers and protecting the public interest, there is a clear bias towards P3s, which is inherent to the very nature of CAMF-dictated decision-making. P3 preference is betrayed, for instance, through the best-practice principle of achieving value for money. Value for money, the CAMF advises, "will be enhanced through strategic use of public and private resources" (ibid.).

Further to the point, the CAMF dictates that any capital project proposal in excess of $50 million must *first* be considered as a P3, although from 2002 to 2008 the threshold was set even lower at $20 million (since 2008 those in the $20–$50 million range are subject to a P3 screen, which is used to determine whether a more comprehensive P3 evaluation should proceed) (BC Ministry of Finance 2008). As Cohn suggests, this shifts the bias away from traditional public procurement by "chang[ing] the terms of debate regarding P3s. Instead of explaining why a P3 was justified, it [is now] necessary to explain why a P3 (or some other form of alternative service delivery) [is] *not* being employed" (2008, 89).

Less obvious but equally important are the implications of its focus on market-oriented notions of risk and the heavy emphasis placed on identifying and valuating risk throughout CAMF procedures. Before a project can move beyond the initial proposal stage, it is subject to a risk-based assessment that privileges the mitigation and minimization of risk through partnership agreements. This fosters an innate bias against public financing and ownership, given that *any* new infrastructure project taken on by a public sector agency that does not involve the private sector is assumed to generate unnecessary risk. Risks are then monetized and added onto publicly delivered projects, penalizing public procurement, even though these risks may be entirely hypothetical. Since risks are expected to be mitigated and minimized, new publicly financed, designed, owned, and operated capital projects are discouraged.

Ontario's Infrastructure Planning, Financing, and Procurement Framework

Initiated in July 2004, Ontario's Infrastructure Planning, Financing, and Procurement Framework (IPFP) is similar to BC's CAMF, given that it outlines the strategies that will be used when developing (planning, building, financing, and managing) new public infrastructure projects across the province. The IPFP was crafted to guide a period of significant, targeted infrastructure renewal. The first phase of this process was the $30 billion ReNew Ontario initiative (2005–10) which "direct[ed] infrastructure investments to the areas that Ontarians have said are their priorities – health care, education and economic prosperity" (Ontario Ministry of Infrastructure 2005). The IPFP continued to guide the subsequent (2011–13) three-year, $35 billion investment plan known as the Building Together initiative, which also targeted important sectors such as health care and transportation. These efforts marked an improvement over previous year-by-year planning and helped to address the significant infrastructure gap in Ontario; however, under the IPFP framework, the process through which investment decisions are made was skewed in favour of P3s.

Much like in BC, the IPFP framework enshrines five key principles in the planning, financing, and approval of project proposals submitted by ministries, municipalities, hospital boards, and other public sector entities. These are: the public interest is paramount, value for money must be demonstrated, appropriate public ownership/control must be preserved, accountability must be maintained, and all processes must be fair, transparent, and efficient (Ontario Ministry of Public Infrastructure Renewal 2004, 9). These are presented as a pragmatic, technocratic approach to infrastructure investment, yet there is an explicit emphasis on "innovative engagement of the private sector to leverage expertise and capital" (17), and P3s must be considered for all projects over $20 million. Of the nine infrastructure and procurement models discussed in the IFPF, eight are P3s (21–2), and the public procurement option is recommended only for very minor investments (24). A risk-focus is present here too, as is an emphasis on value for money.

Risk assessments have therefore come to assume an important role in capital planning in BC and Ontario. Within both provinces, risk identification is integrated at an early stage into capital proposals, and risks are expected to be managed and mitigated. Project risk categories are identical (see table 3).

Table 3. Project Risk (BC and Ontario)

Risk	Example
General	How an initiative fits with established objectives
Policy	How a project might be affected by a change in legislation
Public interest	Health, safety, security, etc.
Management	Team selection, availability of qualified managers, ability to work with private consortia
Design, construction, supplier	Availability of top-quality supplies, contractors, permits obtainable within a suitable timeframe
Site	Site selection: affordability, physical suitability (e.g., soil), possibility of land claims disputes
Financing	Available at the appropriate time, creditworthiness of partners
Cost, economic, market	Any event that could affect cash flow during development
Ownership and operations	Labour relations, maintenance, and technical obsolesce risks
Other	Force majeure

Source: IPRP (Ontario MPIR 2004, 30) and CAMF (BC Ministry of Finance n.d., 18–19).

Beyond these similarities in assessing risk, some important differences begin to emerge. For instance, on the five guiding principles used to inform infrastructure decisions, both provinces share an emphasis on protecting the public interest, achieving value for money, ensuring accountability, and establishing a level of transparency (although along with "transparency" BC emphasizes competition, while Ontario instead emphasizes fairness and efficiency). This leaves one major difference: in BC fiscal management takes precedence, not public ownership or control like in Ontario. This difference, as it relates to provincial P3 programs, constitutes one of the most significant innovations offered by Ontario's Alternative Financing and Procurement model (AFP) (discussed below). In actual practice, however, P3 hospital project agreements in Ontario offer neither greater public ownership nor control – they are structured nearly identically in both provinces. However, it is worthwhile noting that P3 hospital deals initiated in Ontario prior to the AFP model would have allowed for the land and facilities to be owned by the private partner, but under AFP the ownership of the land and facility remains with the public partner. The land and facilities associated with BC's P3 hospital agreements are also publicly owned.

Another major difference between the two capital planning frameworks is that in Ontario risk is associated mainly with infrastructure development and must be considered when conducting assessments of procurement options. Risk for BC is a much broader concept, as it not only encompasses infrastructure procurement but applies to all public sector agencies as well.[6] In BC, whichever public sector agency is "best able" to manage project risks is supposed to take on those responsibilities (BC Ministry of Finance n.d., 9). This accounts for the increased role of the province's dedicated P3 unit, Partnerships BC, with P3 hospital

---

6 Every public sector activity is considered to be inherently "risky," and since 2002 this has meant that ministries and other public sector agencies must undertake Enterprise-Wide Risk Management (ERM) assessments. However, by 2011 the BC auditor general had reported that "government has made insufficient progress in integrating enterprise risk management into its practices despite the official adoption of a risk-based approach in April 2002" (Auditor General 2011b, 6). This has not put a damper on risk-based assessments for P3s, as demonstrated in the government response to the auditor general's report: "While recognizing that implementation to date, on a cross government basis, has not been consistent, ERM has been very successfully used on major projects within government, including all Public/Private Partnership initiatives" (9). Thus risk is the basis of justifying P3s but may be more discursive than actual in other areas.

development (shifting some areas of decision-making away from the regional health authorities and the Ministry of Health). Authority over capital projects is devolved only when a local agency is determined to be low risk, judged in light of its past fiscal and performance targets and track record of past project management. This turns a devolved, region-alized health-management system into a hierarchical system when it comes to capital planning.

In addition, the CAMF holds that risks can be positive and negative, both of which incentivize P3 use. If an agency is unfamiliar with P3s and will be undertaking one for the first time, this carries some degree of risk. However, the CAMF contends that this is a positive risk, given that "a defining feature of P3s is the opportunity they provide to share or transfer risks" (BC Ministry of Finance n.d., 15). Thus P3s are cast as bearers of positive risk (i.e., risks that ought to be taken) and mitigators of negative risk (i.e., through risk transfer to the private sector). It is a win-win situation for the P3 model.

BC's Health Sector Partnerships Agreement Act (Bill 94–2003)

Designed to alter the rights of privatized P3 hospital support staff, BC's Bill 94-2003 (The Health Sector Partnerships Agreement Act) was introduced as a companion[7] to the earlier Bill 29-2002 (The Health and Social Services Delivery Improvement Act), which targeted contracted-out support staff employed in traditional non-P3 hospitals. It has been said of Bill 29, though it could apply equally to Bill 94, that this legisla-tion was introduced for no other purpose but to "provide new invest-ment and business opportunities for private corporations in the health care sector and to reduce compensation for health care support work-ers" (Cohen and Cohen 2006, 117–18). Dispossession was encouraged through both bills, as they allowed for the elimination or alteration of several key provisions in signed collective agreements, namely those that provided job-security protection and protection from privatization, applicable to all "non-clinical" employees in BC's health care sector.

The implications of Bill 94 were not immediate, as BC's first P3 hospital opened several years later in 2006 and the second one later still in 2008, but the effects of Bill 29 were swift and disastrous for non-clinical health care support staff. Within a few short years, more than 9,000 members

---

7 The language and provisions of Bill 94-2003 refer specifically to Bill 29-2002.

of the Hospital Employees' Union had lost their jobs, and wages were slashed and benefits lost in newly contracted-out positions (Cohen and Cohen 2006).

After attempts by union and health care advocacy organizations to challenge Bill 29 through BC courts had failed, the case was brought before the Supreme Court of Canada. In 2007, in a 6–1 ruling, three sections of the legislation were found to be constitutionally invalid: sections 6.2 (no restrictions on contracting-out), 6.4 (no requirement of consultation prior to contracting-out), and 9 (relating to layoffs and bumping). The province was given one year to remedy the situation, and in May 2008 amendments were introduced through Bill 26-2008 (The Health Statutes Amendment Act), which removed those sections from Bill 29 and similar provisions in Bill 94, as they too would have also been vulnerable to the same Charter challenge. However, dispossession-promoting elements of Bill 94 still remain in place. Section 3, for instance, clarifies that the "private sector partner is the true employer" and that a non-clinical staff member is not to be considered "an employee of a health sector partner" (see Bill 94-2003, section 3). Thus Bill 94 allows non-clinical support services provided in P3 hospitals to be privatized and clarifies the nature of this employment: even though they operate within the public health care system, P3 support staff are in fact employees of the private contractor, not the regional health authority. Dispossession in the form of lower wages, fractured bargaining units, and more precarious employment overall have resulted from Bill 29-2002 and Bill 94-2003.

The definition of "non-clinical" in the legislation opens the door to more expanded forms of privatization in the future. Not only does it include support services like laundry, security, housekeeping, and food services, but it also applies to *all* staff except for health services professionals working with patients "admitted to a bed in an inpatient unit in an acute care hospital" (see part 1 in Bill 29-2002; Bill 94-2003 uses its definition of "non-clinical"). In other words, for-profit partners may eventually come to employ most staff working within a P3 hospital. As the BC Nurses' Union warns, "The private consortium could run the hospital emergency room, its rehabilitation beds, day surgeries, outpatient cancer clinics and any other outpatient services for profit. The only services that must be managed under the public health care system would be care provided by nurses and doctors to the sickest patients – those who actually have been admitted to an acute care bed" (BCNU 2003). There has yet to be a P3 hospital project agreement signed in BC that takes advantage of this expanded definition of "non-clinical" in the legislation, but the ability to do so in the future remains nonetheless.

Ontario's Alternative Financing and Procurement Model

ReNew Ontario led to an explosion in the number of P3 hospitals in that province, with nearly forty launched in the first three years alone (Ontario Standing Committee on Government Agencies 2008). Inheriting two yet-to-be-completed projects from the Mike Harris Progressive Conservative government (one in Brampton and one in Ottawa, both announced in 2001), Dalton McGuinty vowed during the election campaign to scrap these plans and assured voters that all hospitals in the province would be owned and operated by the public sector (Blackwell 2003). This promise was not altogether abandoned, as some changes were made to the nature of the ownership agreements of these two initial P3 hospitals, but semantic and procedural differences rather than substantive ones were mainly how it was fulfilled.

Branded a "made in Ontario" solution to a serious infrastructure deficit, P3s in Ontario are now labelled "Alternative Financing and Procurement" (AFP) projects and are subject to the five key principles of the IPFP framework. The "public ownership" and "value for money" principles constitute an improvement over the way previous P3s were developed, as do shorter project agreements and a reassertion of public ownership over land and facilities, yet in practice AFP projects are still P3s. Both models involve partnering with for-profit private consortia for the design, construction, financing, and operation of public infrastructure and support services. P3 industry insiders and advocates also confirm that they see no substantial difference between the two (e.g., see Ontario Standing Committee on Government Agencies 2008, 1530), as did the minister of health when initially presenting AFP to the private sector (e.g., see CCPPP 2005).

However, when comparing BC's health sector P3 program to Ontario's, a clear distinction between AFP and P3 emerges in relation to BC's Bill 94: in 2006 the Ontario Ministry of Health and Long-Term Care decided to exclude what they call "soft support services" from future hospital deals (Sapsford 2006, quoted in Block 2008, 2). This is an important difference between the two programs. Since "soft services" are now distinguished from "hard services" (both of which are classified as "non-clinical" services in BC), recent P3 hospital agreements in Ontario include only facility services like maintenance, security, and operation of the physical plant, exempting care-related services like housekeeping, dietary, and laundry services. Thus there is no legislative counterpart to BC Bill 94 (with its broad classification of "non-clinical services" and its "true employer" provisions) in Ontario.

Why exactly soft services were excluded in Ontario is a multifaceted issue. On one hand, CUPE and the Ontario Health Coalition (OHC) claim that it is the result of a series of community-initiated plebiscites organized by the OHC, which indicated overwhelming community support for the proposition that new hospital projects be kept fully public. A plebiscite in Hamilton, for example, returned a vote of 98 per cent in favour of this proposition (OHC 2006b). From a more critical perspective, soft support services may have instead been exempted as a result of the serious and ongoing problems that have emerged following their incorporation into early P3 hospital project agreements in that province.

The difficulties experienced with managing these contracts is illustrated through a response given by Ken White, former president & CEO of the William Osler Health System (the board that oversees the Brampton P3 hospital, which includes soft support services), when asked about the 2006 exclusion of soft services: "I would say amen to that, actually … these contractual arrangements … are very detailed documents that, first of all, I think are difficult for folks to understand, and it's even more difficult to figure out what measures you want to use to make sure that you're getting the level of service that you need" (Ontario Standing Committee on Public Accounts 2009). It is most likely that this exemption serves both purposes: assuaging public concerns whilst helping to make P3s run more smoothly in the future. By representing both a concession offered to P3 opponents and a pragmatic modification of the P3 model, overall this development has helped ensure the longevity of the P3 program in Ontario's public health care sector.

Supportive Secondary Reforms

The "supportive secondary reform" category encompasses elements of the enabling field that are not essential to P3 project development but are highly supportive reforms specific to particular P3 programs. Within both provincial health sector P3 programs these reforms have shifted responsibility and accountability for certain procedural elements of P3 development to newly created health authorities.

Regional Health Authority Restructuring in BC

The 2001 restructuring of BC's public health management system involved the devolution of authority from the Ministry of Health to new regional health authorities (RHAs) and the simultaneous concentration of power at the regional level (which shifted power away from local health boards, community health councils, and community health societies). The goals of RHA creation were not directly related to P3 promotion but rather were presented as a way to avoid administrative duplication and achieve better regional coordination and greater equity across regions (related to budgets, decision-making, and accountability) (BC Ministry of Health Planning 2002, 2). However, along with these changes came two important P3-related initiatives. First, responsibility for hospital infrastructure planning was given to the RHAs just as budgets were cut (Murphy 2007). This meant that RHAs were suddenly responsible and accountable for tough decisions on service privatization and other "pragmatic" cost-cutting measures, diverting attention from how austerity and dispossession also dovetailed with Cabinet's broader neoliberal policy shift. Second, mandatory three-year performance agreements (known as "service plans") with the Ministry of Health were initiated. Fiscal sustainability and performance became top requirements of these · service plans (BC Ministry of Health Services 2003), as did compliance with the Ministry of Finance's new CAMF capital planning procedures. Together these two changes have all but forced RHAs in need of new infrastructure to seek out private funding via P3s.

Along with new RHAs came new board members appointed by the minister of health. These decision-makers are no longer chosen exclusively for their health care expertise but instead for their business acumen (e.g., see Fraser Health Authority n.d.; Vancouver Coastal Health Authority n.d.). This does not necessarily imply that board members are biased in favour of P3s, but it does facilitate a shift in ethos – from a focus on public service delivery and enhancing health outcomes towards the management of contracts and fiscal performance. This private sector background is also necessary, as RHAs must be increasingly market-oriented and business savvy. RHAs are now responsible for identifying infrastructure needs within their three-year service plans, liaising with other public agencies and private partners during P3 development (throughout all initial stages of a project: bidding, negotiation, construction), and must monitor and enforce performance agreements with private partners during the operational phase of the project (typically thirty years).

Creating Local Health Integration Networks in Ontario

Ontario, unlike most other provinces, has a much more hierarchical health-management structure and has never pursued regionalization. Some restructuring began in 2006 with the creation of geographically based Local Health Integration Networks (LHINs), but actual devolution of authority remains limited as the Ministry of Health and Long-Term Care has retained a significant degree of authority over the LHINs (OHC 2006a). Even though LHINs are responsible for allocating over $20 billion and have the authority to merge services and restructure local health organizations, health-systems experts report that LHINs have been little more than "another layer of unnecessary bureaucracy," and systems improvement has been "throttled by Ministry directives" (Ronson 2011; also see Sullivan and Born 2011). Similar fears, as well as the possibility that they would help facilitate privatization, were expressed by the Ontario Health Coalition in 2006 when the LHINs were first established (OHC 2006a).

LHINs have created a third layer in Ontario's chain of health-system authority, sitting between the hospital boards that govern day-to-day activities within hospitals and the ministry, which sets overarching policy directives and ensures compliance with other Cabinet dictates such as the preference for Alternative Financing and Procurement (AFP). These roles and responsibilities are formalized through performance agreements between the ministry and LHINs, and accountability agreements between LHINs and hospital boards. Despite their disappointing performance in other respects, LHINs indirectly support P3 development, as their administrative expertise helps streamline infrastructure spending and procurement. When a hospital board submits a proposal for new/redeveloped infrastructure valued above $20 million, a LHIN is tasked with helping the board and ministry develop the business case and functional program (Clarke 2010). When a project is valued below $20 million, the LHIN is given far greater autonomy from the ministry and power over the hospital board (Ontario Ministry of Health 2011), but whether this will eventually apply to AFP projects remains to be seen.

New Forms of Institutional Support

New forms of institutional support for P3s are the backbone of the enabling field. The creation of specialized government agencies, or "P3 units," best exemplifies this component. P3 units promote and evaluate

P3s and also act as repositories of knowledge (facilitating policy learning, contract standardization, skill-building, and expertise associated with the complex bidding, negotiation, and the operational phase of P3 projects). The presence of these P3 units has been essential to moving from the development of individual projects to sector-wide programs. There are other organizations that could fit into this institutional support category (e.g., ministry experts, fairness auditors, private consultants), although in BC and Ontario these organizations primarily interact with, or are subsumed by, P3 units, and thus for the sake of simplicity will not be examined here. A more extensive analysis of these P3 units is provided in the chapter that follows.

Partnerships BC

Created in 2002, the Crown corporation Partnerships BC (PBC) acts as a P3 champion, value for money evaluator, and knowledge centre. The last includes developing best practice guidelines and standardizing contracts and bidding processes for future P3s (Rachwalski and Ross 2010). In BC's health sector program this expertise and assistance not only helps with project development but the CAMF also dictates that PBC services must be used for all large hospital projects. Should an RHA propose that a hospital be re/developed within its jurisdiction, the business case must be first forwarded to PBC (and a fee is paid in exchange for the receipt of its specialized services). PBC then analyses the business case to determine which procurement model is best suited for the project (P3 vs traditional). Should the project proceed as a P3, PBC becomes involved in all subsequent stages of development (bidding, contract negotiation, monitoring construction and operations).

There is a serious possibility that PBC, as both evaluator and promoter, is biased towards P3s. Even the World Bank has cautioned that the multiple roles played by PBC may lead to undesirable outcomes (Dutz et al. 2006). PBC denies that a conflict of interest exists (BC Select Standing Committee on Public Accounts 2006); however, the fact remains that since the implementation of the CAMF there has yet to be a single health care infrastructure project valued at over $50 million that PBC has not recommended for development as a full-spectrum DBFO P3 (where the private partner designs, builds, finances, and operates the project), and those in the $20–$50 million range nearly always proceed as design-build P3s (e.g., see Fraser Health Authority 2009; Interior Health Authority 2008).

Infrastructure Ontario

Created in 2005, Infrastructure Ontario (IO) performs many of the same roles as does PBC by evaluating, developing, and creating expertise on P3 implementation in the province. Beyond this, at the level of the P3 health sector program, there are a few differences between the two. First, IO is housed within the Ministry of Infrastructure and thus is not as independent as PBC. Second, IO does not sell its services to hospital boards like PBC does with RHAs; instead it is assigned projects that ministries wish to be developed as P3s. There are many implications that result from these differences but, with respect to how it affects procurement procedures, one worth noting here is that IO becomes involved at a later stage than does PBC. IO does not generally help with infrastructure proposals and business case preparation; this is done through discussions and negotiations among hospital boards, the Ministry of Health, and the relevant LHIN. It is only once a functional program is complete and approved by the ministry that IO becomes involved. After these stages, the differences between the two P3 units become less important, given that under the terms of AFP and IPFP, projects above $20 million are sent to IO for evaluation. IO and the ministry will then initiate P3 bidding, with IO managing and overseeing the entire process. In all but a few instances IO has recommended that projects be developed as P3s (Ontario Standing Committee on Public Accounts 2009), and thus the potential for conflict of interest may mirror the situation in BC.

Concluding Remarks

Initial phase P3s tended to suffer from several fairly high-profile problems such as poor value for money, inadequate risk transfer, community resistance to support-service privatization, loss of public accountability, and other elements related to ill-conceived projects with poorly designed contracts. As a result, early P3 project development in Canada remained highly politicized. By the mid-2000s a second phase had clearly emerged, marked not by a resolution of these problems but instead by an entrenched and much expanded commitment to P3s through the development of sector-wide programs (shifting away from merely developing one-off projects) and the establishment of enabling fields that promote and normalize P3s as the "new traditional."

While enabling field support does not eliminate the pitfalls associated with P3s, it does make them easier to implement, regularizes the process, creates a bias towards privatization; and to the extent that some policy learning takes place then P3s may perform slightly better – or at least appear to. The real significance of the enabling field is thus the way in which it creates a new "common sense," which alters public sector decision-making and procurement processes, leading to more covert and enduring support for privatization when compared with earlier rollback policy (such as Mike Harris's self-styled "Common Sense" revolution in Ontario in 1995). Because P3 policy development now operates at the mundane level of technocratic routines and standardized procedures, concessions can be offered – such as the exemption of soft hospital services from AFP project agreements in Ontario – which represent a victory for P3 opponents while simultaneously improving the longevity of the model. Changes made to P3 development are now done in a controlled fashion, orchestrated largely by P3 proponents and influenced only marginally by opponents of privatization. Further, there is no guarantee that service exemptions will continue indefinitely, nor will dampening dissent do much good for the long-run struggle against dispossession and marketization in the public health care system.

Bob Jessop has characterized neoliberalism as being "ecologically dominant" in the sense that "the profit-oriented market-mediated capitalist economic order taken as a whole – including its extra-economic supports – [is able] to shape other ensembles of social action more than they affect it" (2010, 28). Enabling fields have not yet done for the P3 model what neoliberalism has done for the "profit-oriented market-mediated order," and thus the model is not ecologically dominant even in Ontario and BC. However, inroads of this sort have been made, specifically on large infrastructure projects in these provincial health sectors. For hospital projects, P3s are in many ways the "new traditional" method of procuring goods and services.

The connection between neoliberalism and P3s ought not to be lost in this discussion. Neoliberalism encourages privatization much like enabling fields encourage the selection of P3s over traditional methods. Whether P3s will continue to flourish indefinitely may be impossible to predict, but one thing is certain: their success over the past decade could not have occurred without a reorientation of the public sector's institutions, agencies, and procurement protocols. This makes the items that form an enabling field highly transformative, not merely substitutes for older protocols or ways to fill in gaps that existed with P3 development processes. It is the nature of this transformation – the routinization, institutionalization, and depoliticization of privatization via P3s – that we turn to next.

Chapter 4

P3 Procurement and the Marketization of the Public Sector

The creation of enabling fields in BC and Ontario encouraged the shift to P3s as the de facto standard method of delivering large public infrastructure and support services in those jurisdictions. "Large" refers to those projects where the provincial contribution for construction and equipment is valued at the proposal stage to be in excess of $20 million. The emphasis on "provincial contribution" is important, given that hospital infrastructure (re)development funding often comes from public, private, and third-sector sources.

As discussed in the previous chapter, moving from the development of highly politicized one-off projects in the 1990s and early 2000s to now largely normalized P3 programs within sensitive areas of public policy such as the public health care system relied on a host of new institutional, legal, and capital-planning procedures. This constellation of new arrangements is referred to here as a "P3-enabling field." Enabling fields are more than an amalgam of new policies and institutions; they help rid jurisdictions of the traditional use of public procurement: infrastructure projects that are wholly owned and controlled by the public sector, with contracts awarded to a private for-profit service-provider for a limited and specified role (e.g., construction or laundry services). This has created a new bias towards the P3 model as the standard choice for large capital projects through routinization, institutionalization, and depoliticization (RID).

Routinizing P3 implementation involves normalizing privatization-related policy protocols and developing a familiarity around P3 adoption such that the process is regularized and even rendered mundane. These routines deeply embed the language and calculus of marketized rollout neoliberalism within the heart of public policymaking (marketization being the advancement of market rule and market-like rules within the public sector). Public infrastructure and service decisions are henceforth determined almost exclusively through technocratic, market-oriented procedures: evaluating and monetizing risk, determining value for money, and minimizing upfront capital costs – all of which reorient the "public interest" to favour considerations such as price and risk, even if achieved to the detriment of quality and equity.

Institutionalizing support for P3s further entrenches dispossession and involves the creation of new capital-planning procedures and the empowering of select (sometimes new) public authorities. As an ongoing process, institutionalization also helps create a sense of permanency for P3 policy.

Interrelated with the previous two, the strong popular support exhibited for the public health care system in Canada has meant that initial P3 hospitals were subject to much debate and resistance in the past, and thus depoliticization through the P3-enabling field helps obscure the political nature of dispossession and makes this form of procurement appear as though it is merely a pragmatic decision. Rhetorical forms of depoliticization are also matched by the actual shift from public to private authority that occurs with P3s – making depoliticization both a reality and a strategy.

RID is an ongoing process, not a stationary state. It is "locked-in" through changes and innovations in the P3-enabling field. As an enabling field becomes more sophisticated over time, P3 projects and programs begin to flourish and the model is entrenched, replacing public procurement as the traditional model (for large capital projects in particular). Furthermore, since this process requires policy learning and P3 program evolution, elements of the enabling field may be altered in response to community activism. However, so long as this involves changes made to *how* P3s proceed and not *whether* P3s proceed, adaptations ultimately strengthen the model overall.

Enabling Fields and RID

Once enabling fields were established in Ontario and BC, hospital project proposals that estimated a provincial contribution for construction and equipment in excess of $20 million began to proceed mainly as partnerships with for-profit private consortia. Enabling fields embed accumulation by dispossession within the public sector through the routinization, institutionalization, and depoliticization (RID) of for-profit partnerships with private consortia. Table 4

Table 4. Routinization, Institutionalization, Depoliticization

RID	Description	Features	Examples
Routinization	Capital planning procedures normalize P3 development	P3s become standard practice (the "new traditional") Decision-making focuses on risk, upfront costs, value for money, and a market-oriented notion of the "public interest"	New capital planning procedures • BC's Capital Asset Management Framework (CAMF) • Ontario's Infrastructure Planning, Financing, and Procurement Framework (IPFP)
	Familiarization and regularization of P3 development	Involves the standardization of documents, procedures, and contracts; granting new powers to public authorities charged with promoting P3s	P3 units • Partnerships BC • Infrastructure Ontario New health authorities • BC's restructured regional health authorities (RHAs) • Ontario's Local Health Integration Networks (LHINs)
Institutionalization	The P3 model is entrenched through policy restructuring	New public sector authorities are empowered and/ or co-opted; new modes of decision-making are created	New capital planning procedures • BC's CAMF • Ontario's IPFP • Ontario's Alternative Financing and Procurement (AFP) model P3 units • Partnerships BC • Infrastructure Ontario New health authorities • BC's restructured RHAs • Ontario's LHINs
Depoliticization	The political nature of P3s is obscured, as is the shift towards dispossession and private sector decision-making	Commodification by technocracy is accomplished through routinization and institutionalization	P3 programs • BC Bill 94 • Ontario's AFP model P3 units • Partnerships BC • Infrastructure Ontario New capital planning procedures • BC's CAMF • Ontario's IPFP • Ontario's AFP model

summarizes how some of the examples provided in the previous chapter contribute to RID.

Routinization

Routinizing dispossession within the public sector involves the development and normalization of protocols that facilitate the selection of P3s. There are two important components here: the language of the enabling field (and the entrenchment of risk-based value for money analyses as the primary focus of decision-making) and the normalization of a market-oriented view of how the "public interest" is to be conceptualized and guaranteed. This is accomplished not through grand, ideologically laden offensives but instead through mundane, technocratic procedures.

Given the marketized nature of this form of decision-making, the language of the enabling field is part rhetoric and part reality. The notion that public provision is inherently riskier, more costly since paid for upfront, and of poorer value for money demonizes traditional hospital projects in a way that is reminiscent of the rollback variant of neoliberalism (Peck and Tickell 2002) and first-phase P3 justifications identified by Loxley (2010). For this reason P3 development remains a highly normative process as adherence to, and support for, logics of dispossession require a strong ideological commitment to privatization. However, normative neoliberalism can also work through normalized neoliberal policy (Hay 2004), and that is just what the establishment of routines surrounding P3 selection does. Once normatively based enabling fields are set up and a commitment to developing sector-wide P3 programs is initiated, normalization can proceed through its everyday routines. This indicates that normalized and normative versions of neoliberalism are not mutually exclusive.

Routinization is thus similar to Gramsci's (1971) notion of hegemony, which captures how social norms (in this case, routine capital planning procedures) can foster and cement the dominance of the status quo through the consent of the governed (or here, depoliticize dispossession). The position of P3s as the "new traditional," or status quo, was greatly facilitated by the creation of provincial enabling fields.

Rhetoric is transformed into reality when, as Larner (2000, 33) describes, discourse comes to constitute the institutions and practices of political groups. After a decade or more of developing most large hospital projects as P3s, and of placing an importance on market-based conceptions of risk, the public interest, and value for money, the normative basis of the P3 option is shored up in ways that transcend narrow ideological discourse. This is the essence of what Keil (2009) describes as "rolling with" neoliberalization – when political and economic actors begin to lose a sense of alternatives (good and bad) and thus neoliberal policy becomes self-referential. It is also similar to Peck and Tickell's (2002) description of rollout policy, which is more technocratic and less overtly ideological.

Self-referentiality is a characteristic of P3 policymaking, paradoxically so given that P3 selection remains, on the face of it, justified on the basis of mathematical comparisons made between the P3 and public sector comparator (PSC). However, as the PSC is merely a hypothetical scenario and values alien to marketization (such as a focus on collective decision-making, democratic accountability, and public services *at the expense of* or *without concern for* corporate input, commercial confidentiality, and profitability) are penalized, the role of the PSC is not that of engaging with alternatives to P3s. Rather the biases inherent to P3 value for money analyses (discussed in chapter 2) turn the PSC into a justification for P3 selection. Reinforcing this is the presumption that large infrastructure projects ought to be first considered as a P3. Rolling with neoliberalization in this area of policymaking thus occurs through the language of the enabling field and is reinforced through its processes and routines. Even when improvements are made to overcome past problems with P3s, policy innovations (e.g., standardized contracts and bidding procedures) involve moving the privatization agenda forward.

Institutionalization

An important element in the shift to P3s as the "new traditional" is the institutionalization of this model as the de facto standard way in which large hospital projects are delivered in BC and Ontario. The term "institutionalization" is used here to denote a number of different things. First, the root word – institution – should be taken to literally represent the creation of new public sector agencies (P3 units), which act as centres of expertise for P3 development protocols. Another way to think of institutionalization relates to the way in which new "rules of the game" are formalized through the enabling field and come to shape future decisions, connoting a new system of action and a reorientation of standards and decision-making (see North 1990, 3; Scott 1995, 12). P3 units, new capital planning procedures, and new public agencies tailored to the development of P3s lead to a change in the rules of the game, the norms of the public sector, and the social processes and actions repeated by decision-makers.

An increasing permanence is also denoted by the use of the term institutionalization: these agencies and protocols are no longer expendable and temporary, but are indicative of a marketized regulatory shift. As Selznick states, "Institutionalization is a process ... to 'institutionalize' is to infuse with value beyond the technical requirements of the task at hand" (1957, 16–17). Once P3s begin to proliferate, reference to and experience with previous traditional methods narrow, and the model begins to take on a life of its own (as the "new traditional"). Institutionalization must therefore be conceptualized in process-based terms. In Selznick's description, institutionalization happens to an organization over time, but with the enabling field it is obvious that increasing permanence can also be sped up by the state. In fact both evolution and entrenchment are visible with P3 units and the norms and procedures they embody and reproduce.

This is not to say that processes relating to the evolution of an enabling field are unidirectional and heading ineluctably towards a marketized utopia of P3s as *the* hegemonic model for all public sector engagements. Perhaps a better way of thinking about this category of institutionalization is that it equally encapsulates how different moments of P3 policy are crystallized (i.e., the ways in which challenges are dealt with, created, and absorbed). These challenges come from many directions: neutralizing and accommodating P3 opponents; making good on election promises (or at least appearing to, i.e., AFP in Ontario); dealing with the inherent problems and conflicts associated with privatization, economic/financial crises, and the tendency towards market monopolization; and adjusting to the tensions and trade-offs associated with market-led state restructuring. As Larner argues, "The emergence of new forms of political power does not simply involve the imposition of a new understanding on top of the old ... [it] involves the complex linking of various domains of practice, is ongoingly contested, and the result is not a foregone conclusion" (2000, 20). In other words, P3 development and the "locking-in" of the privatization model is not a foregone conclusion by any stretch; in fact the argument made here is that the whole purpose behind enabling fields and institutionalization is that it provides some semblance of permanency, even though dispossession via P3 requires constant renewal and therefore ongoing political/ideological commitment.

Depoliticization

Depoliticizing privatization policy, or how dispossession is now initiated largely through technocratic decision-making rather than grand normative gestures, is another key implication of the P3-enabling fields in BC and Ontario. Burnham connects depoliticization to a particular governance strategy that "plac[es] at one remove the political character of decision-making" (2001, 127). This benefits state managers by redirecting blame and dampening expectations while still allowing them to retain control. More than merely rhetoric, depoliticization also relies on new bureaucratic practices and a shift from discretion-based to rules-based regimes in particular (Burnham 2001, 130–1). The routines of the new capital-planning and procurement frameworks and P3 units correspond to this conceptualization. It is also suited to describing the larger P3-enabling field as it deals with the internal transformations that occur with state restructuring, indicating that depoliticized decision-making remains simultaneously political.

However, to Burnham's (2001) version of depoliticization (which deals mainly with internal state restructuring) we must add the privatization dimension. Colin Hay (2007, 80–7) provides this in his description of three forms of depoliticization: when issues are demoted from the governmental to the public sphere, from the public sphere to the private sphere, and from the private sphere to the realm of necessity. Depoliticization is thus a process with many faces.

Changes that have occurred with P3s and the creation of enabling fields generally fall within the first two categories of depoliticization. Most obviously, first it involves shifting decision-making from the public sphere into the private sphere. This moment captures the new authority awarded to the private consortia representatives who now influence individual projects, and the private consultants, accountants, and auditors who form the private technocracy that informs policy evaluation. Second, when issues are demoted from the governmental sphere to the public sphere it means that public infrastructure and service decisions are no longer managed primarily through the formal democratic arena (where decision-makers are accountable and public deliberation takes place), but instead are shifted into the far less transparent zone of bureaucratic management (public or quasi-public agencies). This is the realm of the public technocracy, where officials become fairly insulated from public accountability (i.e., P3 units, Local Health Integration Networks, regional health authorities).

Similar to routinization, depoliticization may become a reality in the sense that decisions are shifted into the private sphere, yet it is also remains a powerful rhetorical tactic used by policymakers attempting to duck responsibility for, or reduce the visibility of, privatization. As Ascoli and Ranci (2002, 14) suggest, health sector marketization will always remain politicized, since it "changes the direction in which [health care] policies are developing," making it "an eminently political process, which redistributes rights and power, modifies policy networks and the institutional context in which [health care] policy is made, and influences the ways in which [health care] needs are defined." Furthermore, since hospital infrastructure delivered via a P3 remains a political responsibility (with the public partner ultimately on the hook for funding, procuring, and broadly overseeing the operation of new hospital infrastructure and support services), this form of privatization cannot be truly depoliticized, given that issues are never demoted entirely to the private sphere.

With these three concepts in mind, we turn to a more in-depth examination of how routinization, institutionalization, and depoliticization (RID) are connected to P3 development in BC and Ontario. While all enabling field components identified in the previous chapter play a role in RID, three of the most important elements for P3 hospitals are new capital planning procedures, new/restructured health authorities, and the creation of P3 units in these provinces. Each will be discussed in turn, although all three are highly interrelated in practice.

RID and Capital Planning: Procedures and Authorities

Examining the role of the enabling field focuses attention not only on what is lost (dispossessed) but also on how the neoliberal project restructures states, policy spaces, and protocols, and relies upon the empowerment of new public authorities. The techniques of neoliberalization involve not only grand gestures (overt privatization initiatives) but also the prosaic – the mundane practices and routines through which dispossession is gradually normalized.

Peering into the obscure netherworld of hospital capital planning and procurement illustrates the extent to which routines and new P3-supporting public agencies use market-like rules to make public-policy choices, and the ways in which this decision-making is now a highly technocratic endeavour.

British Columbia

Hospital infrastructure (re)development in BC is composed of two stages: capital planning and implementation (steps and descriptions adapted from the Capital Asset Management Framework Guidelines, see BC Ministry of Finance n.d., 22–59). Five regional health authorities (RHAs) are responsible for identifying needs and ensuring that programs (services and infrastructure) are adequately funded and managed: Vancouver Coastal Health Authority (VCHA), Fraser Health Authority (FHA), Vancouver Island Health Authority (VIHA), Interior Health Authority (IHA), and Northern Health Authority (NHA). A provincial health authority is responsible for province-wide concerns such as cancer care. RHA responsibilities are detailed within three-year service plans, which are agreements between RHAs and the Ministry of Health outlining how responsibilities will be fulfilled.

The service plan lists the goals, priorities, and funding directed to services and infrastructure in that region. It is enforced through performance agreements signed between each RHA and the Ministry of Health, holding the RHA accountable for the how funding is spent. Devolution is not matched by a corresponding increase in discretion surrounding P3 use, this being beyond the control of any particular region. Power has thus been retained by the Treasury (Ministry of Finance) and is influenced in large part by the routines prescribed by the CAMF with its focus on risk identification and monetization, minimizing upfront spending, the P3 screen applied to all large capital spending, and its marketized interpretation of the public interest. Without these routines, decisions made entirely by the premier or at the Cabinet level would remain highly politicized (see the Abbotsford P3 example in chapter 5); and, in contrast, if decisions are made entirely at the regional level, there can be a lack of knowledge and expertise, undermining the normalization of P3 use (see chapter 5 on the Diamond Centre P3).

Table 5 provides a step-by-step breakdown of how hospital infrastructure projects ("capital projects") are planned for and developed in BC, contrasting the NDP-era (1990s) traditional method with the routines of the current P3 health sector program. By creating RHAs and empowering Partnerships BC, along with eliminating the previously institutionalized role for public stakeholder consultations, P3 program decisions made in the initial planning stages are increasingly depoliticized. These decisions have shifted slightly but decisively from the governmental realm to the more opaque realm of the public sector, given that RHAs are one step removed from more politicized governmental decision-making. Accountability to the public is now channelled through the province's Best Practice Guidelines, Governance and Disclosure Guidelines for Governing Boards of British Columbia Public Sector Organizations, and regular (monthly or semi-annual) question-and-answer sessions with the public. The shift

Table 5. BC Capital Planning and Development

Step	Agency		Activity	
	P3 program	Traditional	P3 program	Traditional
1 Identifying local capital needs	RHA	Local agencies*	New capital needs decided on the basis of age/quality of infrastructure, demographics, access, technological change	Consultations with many stakeholders to decide needs
2 Conducting a strategic options analysis	RHA	N/A (traditional procurement bias)	CAMF criteria (cost, risk, complexity, agency track record). P3s must be considered if capital costs exceed $50 million	N/A
	Partnerships BC	N/A	VfM assessment (methodology biased in favour of P3s)	N/A
3 Creating project lists	Ministry of Health	Ministry of Health	Projects are ranked highest if delivered using a P3	Long-Term Capital Plans created by Ministry of Health
4 Constructing Capital Asset Management Plans	Ministry of Health	N/A (similar to step 3)	Forecast of capital asset needs, list of projects that will be used to meet needs	N/A (similar to step 3)
5 Coming up with a Provincial Consolidated Capital Plan	All ministries	Capital division (Ministry of Finance)	Priorities ranked and funding established for all ministry requests	Projects reviewed, submitted to Treasury Board
6 Project approval by Treasury Board	Treasury Board	Treasury Board	If approved, the project is developed through Partnerships BC and by private consortia	If approved, the project is developed mainly by local agencies

(continued)

	Capital Development			
	Agency		Activity	
Step	P3 program	Traditional	P3 program	Traditional
7 Design	Private bidders	Local agencies*	REOI, RFQ, RFP (private design)	Schematic designs prepared, options weighed according to design cost and design value analysis
8 Evaluate, negotiate	Partnerships BC, private bidders	Capital division (Ministry of Finance)	Negotiation of project agreement	Final design approval
9 Project agreement struck (P3), tender (traditional)	Public partner, private partner	Local agencies, private contractor	Private financing, construction, support services	Private construction
10 Implementation	Private partner, public partner Partnerships BC	Local agency British Columbia Building Corporation (BCBC)	Operation, management	Operation, management

Sources: Traditional steps adapted from Deloitte Consulting (2000), P3 program steps taken from BC Ministry of Finance (n.d.)

* BC's Ministry of Health capital planning and funding process prior to 2002 was far more complicated than most. Many "local agencies" were involved, including but not limited to community health councils, community health-service societies, regional health boards, cluster boards, regional hospital districts (and funding agencies), and various associations (e.g., BC Health Association). While the goals of involving a wide range of local agencies may have been lofty – including holding consultations with many stakeholders and ensuring that local planning needs were met simultaneous to provincial health delivery strategies – this approach added a great deal of complexity and ultimately made health capital projects more costly and difficult to complete (the process was much slower and more problems tended to occur along the way, relative to other ministries) (Deloitte Consulting 2000, 5). Some degree of streamlining and restructuring of the traditional capital planning and procurement system was therefore needed; however, the introduction of profit and private decision-making was far from imperative.

in decision-making furthermore indicates a re-conceptualization of the public interest, or at least a transformation in how it is gauged. Depoliticization also takes the form of shifting authority and decision-making into the private for-profit sphere.

Consider the differences presented in the table above, both in incorporating profitability concerns and with the new processes of public sector decision-making that are initiated. Using traditional procurement methods, private for-profit firms are shut out of the infrastructure and service-delivery process almost entirely. Where they are involved, they merely execute the plans and decisions made by the Ministry of Health, Ministry of Finance, and local health authorities. Under the new model, Partnerships BC becomes involved – often as the most important public sector agency, not the agencies normally thought of as responsible for health care: the Ministry of Health and RHA. This infringes upon democratic openness and transparency, as well as accountability. It also ensures that Partnerships BC has a vested interest in P3s, since these projects secure its influence and decision-making position, and are its main source of revenue. It has no role beyond the development of P3s (though it does offer its services outside of BC – more on that later). P3s are therefore a form of marketization in two ways: they allow for direct market rule (private for-profit decision-making) and market-like rules (pushed by the CAMF and Partnerships BC).

Although several roles and responsibilities were devolved to the province's five regional health authorities in 2001, control by the Ministry of Health is ensured through the three-year service plan agreements it holds with each health authority. These commitments outline, among other things, the funding that will be made available from the province for capital project spending in that region. Service plans offer a snapshot of how RID operates at the regional level in BC, since they list all approved capital projects with a cost of over $2 million. Reviewing these agreements (see FHA 2009, 2011; IHA 2011; NHA 2010; VCHA 2010; VIHA 2010) produces some interesting results.

First, P3s are being institutionalized through the routines and rules established by the CAMF, given that *all* capital projects with an estimated cost in excess of $50 million are now going forward as P3s. Said another way, no capital project that could have been delivered as either a P3 or in the traditional public fashion will be a public project. P3s are now the standard model for large hospital infrastructure development in the province. This indicates a high level of P3 institutionalization.

What is occurring with the projects that fall within the grey zone of costing between $20 and $50 million is equally informative. In 2012, seven hospital re/development projects were listed in the five RHA service plan agreements, with costs ranging from roughly $23 million to $44 million.[1] None are being developed as DBFO P3s, but few are being delivered through in-house tender either (the truly "traditional" version of a hospital project) – most are design-build P3s and not listed on the PBC website, under-representing the degree to which bundled for-profit contracts are a feature of the BC capital development landscape. Those that are fully public (e.g., both Vancouver General Hospital projects in the Vancouver Coastal Health Authority) are those closest to the $20 million threshold and have received sizable contributions from third-sector sources (donations to hospital foundations and auxiliaries).

The language and risk emphasis of the CAMF also favours P3 use. One of the key objectives of the CAMF is to link RHA needs with provincial policy priorities. This embeds a P3 bias into decision-making early on, and risk-based assessments (using value for money and other technocratic criteria) are relied on to gauge whether RHA needs match up with CAMF dictates. Since risks must be minimized, and this is to be accomplished by keeping upfront costs down, the public role in new infrastructure must be kept to a minimum.

Furthermore, the public interest is now to be determined primarily through marketized criteria such as assessing service outcomes (through monetization) and monitoring the performance of service-providers (through market-based contracts containing performance agreements). In order to do so, commodification of health care support services and a reorganization of tasks within hospitals must first occur.[2] The public interest is also "ensured" through the caveat that service-users must be protected (i.e., user fees may not be applied to medically necessary services protected by the Canada Health Act). No protection is offered against commercialization and the establishment of for-profit

---

1 FHA: Surrey Memorial Hospital Site Immediate Capacity Development, $26 million, Chilliwack General Hospital Redevelopment, $35 million; IHA: Coronary Revascularization Transition Plan, $21 million; VCHA: St Mary's Hospital Redevelopment total project, $44 million, Vancouver General Hospital Robert H.N. Ho Research Centre, $39 million; Vancouver General Hospital Tertiary Mental Health – window pavilion, $29 million; VIHA: Nanaimo Regional General Hospital Emergency Department / Psychiatric Emergency Service / Psychiatric Intensive Care Expansion, $37 million; NHA: no capital projects with a value of $20–50 million in 2012.
2 See Armstrong and Armstrong (2010, 160–2) for a description of how neo-Taylorist techniques have been introduced into hospitals in order to control ancillary workers and reduce the costs of support services.

clinics within P3 hospitals. The public interest is conflated with access and cost sustainability in an immediate sense – there is little concern demonstrated for the long-term implications that might result from higher costs over the life of the project, the potential for trade agreement disputes, and service quality deterioration. This is a very narrow conception of the public interest.

Ontario

The stages that major capital projects (hospital planning and development) are subject to in Ontario, and the respective roles played by the various public and private sector agencies are summarized in table 6.

The procedures in Ontario differ somewhat from those in BC for several reasons, primarily as a result of the difference in public authority structures (within the health sector and for the P3 unit), not the criteria used to evaluate proposals/business cases, despite AFP being touted as fundamentally different from P3. Since Ontario does not have a regionally devolved decision-making structure within its provincial health care system, the MOHLTC has retained more formal control and decision-making authority over P3 development than is the case in BC (although, as was presented above, Ministry of Health guidelines control RHAs in a similar way). However, some administrative functions have been assigned to Local Health Integration Networks (LHINs), and hospital boards play an initial role in infrastructure planning and service-needs identification. As discussed in the previous chapter, the roles and responsibilities of each level of decision-making are formalized through performance agreements struck between the ministry and LHINs and accountability agreements between LHINs and hospital boards.

The emphasis on minimizing risk and addressing needs through options determined using market-oriented value for money assessments is similar in Ontario and BC. The strong cost-savings language in BC is not present in Ontario's IPFP, however. Whatever the justification, in Ontario, hospital infrastructure projects with construction and equipment costs in excess of $20 million are all now being delivered through a P3,[3] and projects under this threshold typically go forward as

---

3 However, in Ontario P3 hospital projects can vary quite widely in type, from build-finance to design-build-finance-maintain. In BC, P3 hospital projects are most often design-build-finance-operate.

Table 6. Ontario Capital Planning and Development

Step	Agency	Activity
	Initial Stages (AFP and traditional follow the same path)	
1 Infrastructure planning needs assessment	Public hospital board (service portion may be assessed with LHIN)	New capital needs decided on the basis of age/quality of infrastructure, demographics, access, technological change
2 Proposal	LHIN, Ministry of Health and Long-Term Care (MOHLTC)	Hospital board submits a description of the program and service elements of a capital initiative to the LHIN for review. If approved by the LHIN, the hospital board provides an estimate and description of the physical elements and capital costs to the MOHLTC
3 Functional program development	Hospital board, LHIN, MOHLTC	With MOHLTC support, the hospital board and its integrated consultant team prepare the function program, outlining the size and scope of the project. LHINs are responsible mainly for ensuring that infrastructure plans match service needs in the region. MOHLTC ensures submissions are consistent with government priorities and that alternative infrastructure delivery options are provided
4 Functional program analysis	MOHLTC, Ministry of Infrastructure	Procurement alternatives are assessed.* This takes place before a project is assigned to Infrastructure Ontario and AFP value for money assessments (if cost exceeds $20 million)

Advanced Stages (AFP and traditional follow different paths)

Step		Agency		Activity	
AFP	Traditional	AFP	Traditional	AFP	Traditional
1 Preliminary design development	Preliminary design development	Infrastructure Ontario, MOHLTC	MOHLTC	Schematic design and transaction documents are developed. Using AFP guidelines, Infrastructure Ontario conducts a value for money (VfM) assessment	In-house design development (block schematic report, sketch plan report)
2 Contract development	RFP, commercial close and financial close	Infrastructure Ontario, hospital board (RFP stage), private bidders	MOHLTC, hospital board	Private design, VfM assessments (prior to contract, after financial close), negotiation of project agreement	In-house working drawings, final cost estimates, procurement (construction contract)
3 Implementation	Implementation	Private partner, public partner, Infrastructure Ontario	MOHLTC, hospital board	Private financing, construction, support services	Public infrastructure (MOHLTC), public services and infrastructure maintenance (hospital)

Source: Adapted from Barrett and Hodnett (2010); Clarke (2010); LHIN (2010); Ontario MPIR (2004). See also: Ontario Auditor General 2014, 194–5.

* The strategic options analysis involves nine models, ranging from fully public (traditional) to design-build-own-operate (DBOO) P3s. Criteria include financial considerations, risk assessments, and value for money calculations, but also emphasize a context assessment for different sectors. Health care projects must engage community and key stakeholders and feature public ownership, control, and accountability (Ontario MPIR 2004, 27). The Ministry of Infrastructure is involved mainly as a way of ensuring that infrastructure financing and procurement follow the IPFP criteria (risk-based, value for money assessed, upfront costs minimized), and it provides direction on the procurement approach chosen.

traditional projects (falling under different capital-planning procedures known as the Health Infrastructure Renewal Fund guidelines).

A clearer attempt to ensure public ownership and control over hospital P3s is present with Ontario's IPFP and AFP (in contrast to BC's CAMF), but guidelines offer no guarantee. In addition, the same concerns with the market-oriented conception of the public interest in BC are present in Ontario. There are a few differences in the role of the P3 unit in each province, although these are best dealt with in the section that follows (which looks at RID and P3 units).

Prior to the development of the P3-enabling field in Ontario, the Harris Progressive Conservative government initiated some important capital planning changes worth highlighting, as they further indicate the degree of RID attained under Liberal governments since 2003.[4]

Whereas the Common Sense Revolution of the Harris government's first term (1995–9) corresponds quite strongly to rollback neoliberalism, the second term (1999–2003) saw a softening of this "revolutionary" emphasis and thus began some attempts at rollout neoliberal policy aimed at normalizing P3 development. Most notably this includes commitments made to greater infrastructure spending, the creation of a public sector agency with features resembling those of a contemporary P3 unit, attaching guiding principles to public spending, and the reorganization of capital planning procedures. However, as the short description below reveals, these initiatives did not lead to routinization, institutionalization, or depoliticization; nor did they constitute a sophisticated enabling field.

In 1999 the Harris government launched a five-year, $20 billion infrastructure spending plan, known as the SuperBuild initiative, which aimed to address the growing provincial infrastructure deficit (Ontario SuperBuild Corporation 2000, 6). Infrastructure needs were to be met through both public and private financing and the use of P3s, under the strategic direction of the newly created Cabinet Committee on Privatization and SuperBuild (CCOPS). These SuperBuild funds were to be distributed and managed by the SuperBuild Corporation (created in 2000), an agency that reported to the Ministry of Finance and deputy premier. The SuperBuild Corporation was responsible for P3 and capital infrastructure strategies province-wide (including providing expertise to other public sector agencies).

---

4 There were no infrastructure P3s developed, and no significant attempts to establish a P3-enabling field in BC prior to 2002, making this type of comparison impossible for that province.

Three principles guided the SuperBuild Corporation's activities: the agency was to facilitate joint public-private investments in infrastructure, to reorient capital-planning procedures and priorities, and to ensure that investment decisions brought the best value to taxpayers and highest returns to private partners (Ontario SuperBuild Corporation 2000, 6–7). SuperBuild was to report all spending and capital recommendations to the CCOPS – creating a unique decision-making structure, given that "for the first time in Ontario, all provincial infrastructure policy, investment and capital planning decisions [were] consolidated under a single Cabinet committee" (6). Two P3 hospitals were initiated in this fashion – the Brampton Civic Hospital and the Royal Ottawa Hospital – but they had entered only the early planning stage by the 2003 provincial election.

Prior to the reorganization of capital-spending and planning procedures under the CCOPS, the process followed a traditional route similar to the one described above for BC (see Ontario Ministry of Health 1996): the hospital board identified capital needs and sought MOHLTC approval for all proposals, options, plans, funding, design, and tendering stages. If approved, the hospital board was responsible for executing and managing these stages. For its part, the MOHLTC was given its own capital funds by government and set its own list of priorities for distributing these funds. SuperBuild changed this arrangement by requiring that all capital plans be sent for approval to the CCOPS before the ministry received any funding for infrastructure (re)development (Ontario SuperBuild Corporation 2000, 8).

SuperBuild was similar to Infrastructure Ontario in that it was to be a centre of expertise on P3s and was positioned to be the evaluator of P3 proposals. It also signalled the beginning of an institutionalized partnership program. However, the CCOPS process was highly politicized (located within Cabinet itself), and SuperBuild was never designed to be an arm's-length decision-maker. There was also no effort made to initiate the routinization seen with the technocratic procedures of the IPFP process developed under the McGuinty government. Finally, the more pragmatic principles of AFP (such as three value for money assessments, greater transparency and more effective risk transfer, public ownership of hospital sites and facilities, and the $20 million P3 threshold) stand in contrast to the opaque SuperBuild decision-making process that was rhetorically (and intentionally) biased towards short-term cost savings, maximizing private returns, leveraging private investment, and developing as many P3s projects as possible. As a testament to the importance of RID and the Liberals' P3-enabling field, SuperBuild produced only a handful of highly controversial deals (e.g., the sale of Highway 407 and the twenty-year Bruce Power nuclear power plant lease) and "the very few deals that have worked as the model envisaged have been small projects" (McFarland 2001).

RID and P3 Units

P3 units have played a crucial, if not the most important, role in routinizing, institutionalizing, and depoliticizing P3 use (RID). They are the primary public sector agencies charged with promoting P3 projects and overseeing project agreements. The encouragement of RID by these agencies is achieved indirectly through the support they offer for the capital procurement routines that privilege P3s and the health authorities (provincial and local/regional) that must follow these protocols. Support is also directly provided through the role played by P3 units in standardizing documents, bidding procedures, and contract development.

New Public Sector Capacity: Commonalities and Particularities

New forms of institutional support for P3s are the backbone of any sophisticated P3 program. P3 units promote and evaluate these projects and act as repositories of knowledge that facilitate policy learning by building government expertise surrounding the complex bidding, negotiation, and operational phase of P3 projects (Rachwalski and Ross 2010). The presence of these P3 units has been essential to the entrenchment and normalization of privatization within the public sector. Yet the role of the P3 unit extends beyond the activities outlined on their websites and in policy documents, as they must translate policy models and neoliberal privatization imperatives, ensuring that this unfolds in ways that meet local needs whilst simultaneously ensuring profitability for global investors.

Without the institutional support that P3 units provide, problems experienced with individual projects would not readily transform into a sophistication of provincial P3 programs and instead could easily lead to policy abandonment. As discussed in chapter 1, P3s are distinct from other types of privatization. Whereas individual projects are locked in through multi-decade contracts, the program itself must be future-oriented, since it is renewed only through new projects. Committed policymakers must therefore take into consideration the long-run implications of decisions made today. P3 units are currently the central way to ensure that this happens. As Jooste and Scott (2012, 150, emphasis added) put it, "The move toward private participation in infrastructure does not simply substitute private sector capacity for public sector capacity, *it requires new forms of public sector capacity to be developed to overcome [P3] challenges."*

The need for new forms of public sector capacity to facilitate internal privatization was resolved in BC and Ontario through the creation of Partnerships BC and Infrastructure Ontario (in 2002 and 2006, respectively), both of which are Crown corporations. This organizational form is significant, given that in some countries greater political control is retained through the development of expertise and P3 unit-like roles within line departments (e.g., Mission d'Appui aux PPP in France and Parapublica in Portugal; see Farrugia, Reynolds, and Orr 2008). On the opposite end of the spectrum, many of the activities performed by P3 units can also be provided by private fairness auditors, consultants, and accountants.

The use of Crown corporations, an arm's-length quasi-public organizational form, has a long history in Canada and they have been assigned many different purposes, ranging from economic development to cultural preservation (Whiteside 2012). Yet something entirely new appears to have occurred in the past decade with P3 units: the use of Crown corporations to facilitate dispossession. This occurs not through their sale but through their very existence – they are developed by the state to manage and encourage privatization in other areas of the public sector. Thus the Crown corporation is now being employed to extend market-led restructuring within Canada's public sector.

The monopolization of support roles required to deal with P3 problems by arm's-length public agencies (rather than being shared with line departments or the private sector) improves the longevity of the P3 model for several reasons, all of which relate to RID. First, it lends itself to depoliticization since they appear to represent the public interest and fall under the direction of government but are free from a high degree of public scrutiny and control. Thus P3 units are at best *quasi*-public agencies. A related consideration is that P3 units clearly serve the interests of capital. As former PBC president and CEO Larry Blain so aptly described, "There are two sides to a [P3] market. There is the province, which has an interest in procurement on an effective and least-cost basis. There is also the private partners who need to be interested in British Columbia and want to do business here and want to do business with us [PBC]. We have to attract them, so we have to attract both sides ... that's our role" (BC Select Standing Committee on Public Accounts 2006).

Second, as Crown corporations they are able to offer salaries and bonuses that often exceed normal bureaucratic pay scales and opportunities. Higher salaries and bonuses for those employed by P3 units mean that private sector business leaders and P3 industry insiders can be more easily recruited into the public sector. For example, in 2005 president and CEO of PBC Larry Blain earned $519,448 in salary and bonuses (bonuses being tied to the number of P3s developed). These exorbitant earnings for a "public sector" employee, along with revelations that taxpayer-funded reimbursements for expenses included, for example, a 23 June 2005 restaurant bill for $1,567.11, created a minor scandal in BC when the figures were eventually made public in 2006 (see Macleod 2007). When pressed to account for this level of compensation, finance minister Carole Taylor claimed Larry Blain's compensation was justified on the grounds that it was necessary "to bring someone with tremendous financial experience in the private sector into the public sector" (Francis 2006). Compensation for upper-echelon decision-makers within Infrastructure Ontario is slightly more modest. For instance, those holding positions such as executive vice-president and CEO earn roughly $330,000–$375,000 – in line with similar positions in Crown agencies like the Ontario Energy Board, but nearly triple the amount of most other publicly disclosed public sector salaries (Ontario Ministry of Finance 2012).

Another feature relevant to institutionalization is a creeping expansion of the roles played by these P3 units. For PBC, expansion has been both internal and external to the province. Internally, the development of P3 programs in key sectors targeted for provincial infrastructure renewal has meant that PBC has been gradually taking over the roles previously played by the BC Building Corporation (BCBC) (McKellar 2006). Thus BCBC, the public sector agency responsible for real estate, land, and infrastructure management since 1977, is being incrementally replaced with a market-oriented quasi-public Crown corporation geared towards privatization. PBC has also become more externally oriented. As indicated in its 2011 annual report (PBC 2011), PBC's future strategy includes diversifying its client base. This involves selling its expertise to other jurisdictions without P3 units (e.g., Yukon and Nova Scotia, see "NDP Questions" 2005; Government of Nova Scotia 2008) and expanding into new sectors within the province (see table 7).

The roles assigned to Infrastructure Ontario (IO) have also been greatly expanded over the years, and it is now responsible for many different aspects of infrastructure and land development in the province: from large P3 infrastructure development and operation beginning in 2005 to small infrastructure loans (offered to municipal borrowers only) as of 2006 when it absorbed the Ontario Strategic Infrastructure Financing Authority (OSIFA), and more recently in 2011 it took on the responsibilities of the Ontario Reality Corporation (ORC) (the manager of

Table 7. Partnerships BC Work Fees

	$			% of PBC revenues		
	2011	2010	2009	2011	2010	2009
Ministry of Health Services and provincial health authorities	1,908,576	2,205,279	2,948,454	22.7	33.2	42.4
Ministry of Transportation and Infrastructure	1,919,946	1,475,085	1,196,532	22.8	22.2	17.2
Ministry of Labour and Citizens' Services	665,465	472,888	426,005	7.9	7.1	6.1
Ministry of Education	520,763	314,745	176,815	6.2	4.7	2.5
BC Crown corporations	1,731,669	462,895	177,980	20.6	7.0	2.6
BC vocational institutes	98,741	301,180	741,944	1.2	4.5	10.7
Other provincial governments	36,876	215,305	220,395	0.5	3.2	3.2
Government of Canada	657,037	706,284	614,976	7.8	10.6	8.8
Others	865,698	498,302	453,711	10.3	7.5	6.5
Total	8,404,771	6,651,963	6,956,812	100.0	100.0	100.0

Sources: PBC (2010, 22; 2011, 20)

government-owned and occupied land and buildings) (see Infrastructure Ontario 2011). This has not only given IO greater degree permanence within the province but it also means that its P3-specific tasks are ever more normalized within the day-to-day operations of government.

But along with similarity comes particularity. A major divergence between these two P3 units is where they are located within the public sector: PBC reports only to the Ministry of Finance, whereas IO falls under the purview of the Ministry of Infrastructure. This relates to a second difference: PBC is far more autonomous and entrepreneurial than IO, as Ontario's P3 unit remains more tethered to government. For instance, IO is assigned projects by line-ministries, and its operations are paid for out of the Ministry of Infrastructure's[5] budget (for budget expenditures related to IO, see Ontario Ministry of Finance 2009). PBC, on the other hand, must generate its own business and touts its operations

---

5 Since the creation of IO in 2005, this ministry has been also named the Ministry of Energy and Infrastructure and the Ministry of Public Infrastructure Renewal.

as being "self-sustaining," since it acts almost entirely independent of government funding by charging "work fees" in exchange for its services (PBC 2011). However, "work fees" are better thought of as a hidden drain on the budgets of other ministries, given that this acts as a way of funnelling money into PBC coffers. The fees it receives are substantial, as table 7 indicates. Note that the Ministry of Health and regional health authorities are the single largest contributor, as a result of the large number of hospitals and health care–related P3s initiated since 2002.

Besides transferring funds from in-house ministry project development to PBC project development, an additional concern with PBC's work fees is the potential for a conflict of interest to exist, given that this P3 unit both evaluates and promotes P3s. As Colverson indicates, "If a dedicated unit is not wholly funded by the government and derives part of its income through user fees it charges there is a risk that P3s can be pushed into inappropriate situations because the unit will have a vested interest in producing business" (2012, 14). Larry Blain denies that this warning applies to PBC, saying, "Part of our [PBC] mandate and our vision statement is that we serve the public interest. We are owned by the province of British Columbia, and part of our mandate is to serve the public interest. We would be sensitive to that in everything that we do" (BC Select Standing Committee on Public Accounts 2006).

A few additional procedural differences worth noting are that IO reimburses the design and bid fees incurred by unsuccessful consortia that make it past the RFP stage, whereas PBC does not do this. PBC has also created an important role for privatized aspects of the enabling field, private fairness auditors in particular.

Failing Forward: Flanking and Deepening (Concessions and Co-option)

Bob Jessop (2002) argues that neoliberalism and the social, economic, and political problems that it creates require flanking by other non-neoliberal strategies such as neo-statism and neo-corporatism. In his words, "Governance has always depended upon a contradictory balance between marketized and non-marketized organizational forms" (238). This insight dovetails with Tickell and Peck's (2003, 165) discussion of how neoliberal market politics have always been hybrid – never appearing in "pure" form, local neoliberalisms are the result of the balance of class forces, institutional legacies, and modifications in light of resistance, path dependency, and crises. Thus we are alerted by both of these perspectives to be on the lookout for unevenness and local particularities, conditions that are generated especially in light of the internal and external problems produced by neoliberal reforms. Peck (2010, 6, 21–3) calls this "failing forward": despite the regulatory inadequacies of neoliberal policy, failures lead not to the abandonment of neoliberalism but to their deepening and complexification through concessions, exceptions, and corrections. With provincial P3 hospital programs, flanking and deepening are best exemplified through the creation of, and actions of, P3 units.

It is crucially important to remember that P3 projects are not developed by P3 units tabula rasa. They unfold within the context of interaction and comparison with real and hypothetical models of traditional infrastructure projects. This comparison (at the heart of establishing value for money) is in fact one of the main features that drives the selection of P3s over public hospitals by PBC and IO. This dichotomy both justifies P3s and presents continual challenges to future P3 development: it offers the potential for crises of faith to occur, allows for overt failures to emerge, forces hard questions, fans the flames of resistance, and can ultimately strengthen the P3 model by forcing adaptation and concessions. The issue of stabilization amid P3 project and policy contradictions will be returned to in the concluding chapter.

RID and Enabling Fields: Four Themes

Four themes emerge when examining P3-enabling fields and their routinizing, institutionalizing, and depoliticizing effects:

1 The creation of new P3-oriented agents, institutions, and procedures suggests that state restructuring and reorientation have occurred, not merely that one form of project procurement is being substituted for another. It also indicates that P3 markets in Canada are well beyond the experimentation stage. Institutionalization proceeds without any systematic effort to evaluate P3 model success in either jurisdiction. Hence the policy is mainly ideologically driven rather than being empirically based, as proponents most often suggest.

2 There are many similarities and differences between enabling fields in Ontario and BC, and thus while there may be a global trend of P3 proliferation, jurisdictions and processes remain variegated and locally particular. RID flourishes amid, and in spite of, differences between enabling fields.

3 Both flanking and deepening are occurring. The former refers to the elements of state restructuring that contribute to dispossession

(i.e., the adoption of market-like rules and routines by the state), and the latter captures how P3s are transformed into the "new traditional" through token concessions made to opponents, modifications of the P3-enabling field, and ultimately the insulation of the P3 model from crises of faith among policymakers through institutionalization.

4 Pragmatism (e.g., the $20 million threshold) and sophistication (e.g., contract and bidding standardization, AFP) are important developments in Canadian P3 policy, given that dislocations and controversy are better absorbed when enabling fields are present. This helps to shore up the P3 model overall and means that the benefits of enabling field innovation are captured mainly by investors not by service users, labour, or taxpayers.

Concluding Remarks

P3s are a form of ongoing and future-oriented dispossession. Their recent proliferation has been pre-staged by a number of legal-institutional and policy supports that operate both as flanking mechanisms (Jessop 2002) and as a way of embedding market-enhancing strategies within the heart of public policymaking. Deepening the influence of market actors and market-based reasoning has meant forging enabling fields out of a hybrid combination of pre-existing and novel institutional/regulatory arrangements through P3-oriented routines and institutions. Enabling fields both subsume and transform pre-existing bureaucratic processes and lead to depoliticization (both real and rhetorical).

The routinization, institutionalization, and depoliticization of P3s is therefore an ongoing process, not a stationary state. RID is "locked-in" through various changes and innovations, including legislative changes and new capital-planning procedures, supportive secondary frameworks as indirect support for P3s, and new institutions/government agencies. Together these changes enable P3s to move from being one-off projects to the new norm for large infrastructure development and its accompanying support services.

Nothing presented here should be taken to suggest that jurisdictions without enabling fields are not, or have not been, developing P3s. Whether at the provincial or municipal level, most provinces in Canada have developed at least one P3, although outside of BC and Ontario these efforts have been sporadic and the focus thus far has been limited mainly to developing projects, not programs (Quebec and Alberta may be shifting to a program focus). At the federal level there are also several operational

P3s, and the Harper Conservatives have implemented a P3 screen (applicable to all funding through the Building Canada initiative) and a P3 unit (PPP Canada). However, as a result of the constitutional division of powers, the sectors with projects that have thus far proven most suitable for partnership agreements are located mainly within provincial jurisdiction (e.g., hospitals, schools, highways, water-treatment facilities).

Furthermore, the argument made here is not that enabling fields unequivocally force ministries and other public authorities to choose the P3 procurement model. Instead what enabling fields do, as the name would suggest, is *enable* P3s by simplifying processes, and encouraging, supporting, and promoting their use. "Enable" may be an understatement, as some items do compel public authorities to consider P3s (i.e., CAMF and IPFP), and even the more coercive items are mere frameworks that could be easily altered, transcended, or ignored if there was the political will to do so. Rather it is the sheer bulk of the enabling field and all of its constituent categories (enabling legislation and new capital-planning frameworks, supportive secondary reforms, and new institutions) that act as a form of soft lock-in by shifting the bias away from traditional public procurement. Soft lock-in also helps depoliticize these activities, just as P3s themselves depoliticize dispossession through technocratic decision-making.

Enabling fields may also help P3 programs weather crises, whether the crisis is economic or political. From a value for money perspective, as examined in chapter 2, we have recently seen the insulating effects of enabling fields when the serious problems with the private finance portion of early-stage P3s in 2008/9 led only to minor changes in P3 programs (e.g., the use of a "wide equity" model in BC). Politically, though this has not yet been tested in BC and Ontario, should an election bring a change in government, institutionalization may lead to policy inertia and thus dissuade P3 program abandonment.

Whether lock-in has occurred or will occur is of utmost significance to the study of privatization policy. A greater understanding of how exactly dispossession now proceeds within the public sector allows for resistance to be made more effective. Just as how P3 promoters have shifted their focus from projects to programs, the organizations and actors that hope to eliminate privatization from the public health care system must too. Targeting individual P3s is one way to do so, but with enabling fields left untouched these efforts will likely be of limited success.

Chapter 5

British Columbia's Pioneering P3 Hospitals

BC's first two P3 hospitals (in Abbotsford and Vancouver) were also among the first P3 hospitals developed in Canada, and they offer many insights into P3 hospital projects, health sector privatization, and the importance of enabling fields in the normalization of P3 use. The hospital projects examined in this chapter were developed at the same time as the provincial enabling field and thus before routinization, institutionalization, and depoliticization (RID) had truly begun. For this reason they are exceptionally revealing. Cast as "pilot" projects by the Liberal government in the early 2000s, they were not used, as one might assume, to establish whether the P3 model had a place in future BC hospital development but rather to launch a P3 program in the health sector. However, this first round of P3 hospital projects lacked the well-honed routines, institutional support, and established forms of depoliticization that now shape the program. The cases examined here reveal the significant effort that went into normalizing health sector marketization and dispossession and clearly indicate the economic, financial, and social implications that enabling fields and RID have attempted to ameliorate, suppress, and ignore ever since. The appendix should also be consulted for its detail on the timeline and milestones of each hospital project.

Initiation: BC's Pioneering P3 Hospitals

The emergence of private for-profit P3 hospitals in BC began with the Abbotsford Regional Hospital and Cancer Care Centre in 2003 (operational in 2008) and the Diamond Centre[1] in 2002 (operational in 2006). Both facilities were sorely needed. The new hospital in Abbotsford replaced an older, rundown, and inadequate hospital in the region, and the Diamond Centre allowed for the reconfiguration and consolidation of existing facilities as a way of improving teaching and training done by the University of British Columbia and patient access to ambulatory services provided by the Vancouver General Hospital. By 2012, another eight P3 hospital and health-centre projects had been launched across the province, and these two pioneers were commonly seen at the time to be a "proving ground" for the P3 model in the health sector (e.g., McInnes 2003). Yet despite the obvious need for each facility, the use of a P3 to deliver this infrastructure and its support services was far from imperative. Instead their development demonstrates the highly political nature of P3s, rather than being, as is too often suggested, the product of financial necessity or clear value for money superiority.

Background

In May 2001, the Liberal party won a landslide victory, taking seventy-seven of seventy-nine seats in the provincial legislature and ousting the two-term NDP government that had held power since 1991. With this victory came a great many changes in government policy and practice, P3s being but one part of the neoliberal flowering that ensued. Infrastructure DBFO P3s of the sort that had been used for nearly a decade in the United Kingdom had popped up here and there across Canada but had not yet been attempted in BC. The NDP introduced the language of P3s in 1997 when the minister of finance said, in a Budget speech, "We are also committed to pursuing public-private partnerships that allow for cost-effective solutions to developing and financing new facilities" (BC Liberal Party 2009), and in 1999 the NDP released a document that counselled municipalities on the (potential) advantages

---

1 Originally the project was called the Academic Ambulatory Care Centre, then renamed the Gordon and Leslie Diamond Centre in 2006, when the Diamonds donated $20 million to "fund state-of-the-art medical equipment at the new centre, establish a new Leslie Diamond Fund for Women's Health, expand the women's and men's urological health program and help provide funding for a new CT scanner for the emergency department at Vancouver General Hospital" (Campbell 2006). This portion of the hospital's redevelopment does not relate in any way to the P3 deal (it was established for separate purposes), yet since that is the name of the new centre, here the P3 will be referred to as such.

of partnering with the private sector (BC Ministry of Municipal Affairs 1999), but these two relatively minor items had amounted to little by 2001. Privatization was not a major feature of the BC policy landscape, and there were only a handful of small municipal P3s that were mainly support-service-related. This would change dramatically after the 2001 election.

Having campaigned under their "New Era" banner of prosperity through fiscal prudence, reinventing government, and creating private sector investment opportunities, the Liberal government quickly began a process of simultaneous neoliberal rollback and rollout. The most important rollout reforms relevant to P3 development are the items that formed the enabling field – especially the 2002 creation of Partnerships BC and the Capital Asset Management Framework. Rollback reforms included Bill 2-2002 (The Health and Social Services Delivery Improvement Act) and Bill 94-2003 (The Health Sector Partnerships Agreement Act). Both bills were designed to "provide new investment and business opportunities for private corporations in the health care sector and to reduce compensation for health care support workers" (Cohen and Cohen 2006, 117–18). This legislation allowed for the elimination or alteration of several key provisions in signed collective agreements, namely those that provided job-security protection and protection from privatization (discussed in greater detail later in this chapter). Corporate and personal income taxes were also slashed immediately following the Liberal victory, including an across-the-board 25 per cent cut to personal income tax – the government's largest source of revenue (Cohn 2006). This seriously undermined the government's main source of revenue and was subsequently used to justify the need for greater private financing of public infrastructure (ibid.).

Along with the decisive Liberal majority came opportunism as high-profile, much-needed infrastructure projects were targeted for the unfolding of its P3 agenda. These efforts zeroed in on the transportation and health sectors, four prime examples being the currently operational Sea-to-Sky highway, Canada Line, and the two hospitals that will be examined shortly. But it must also be noted that there were equally high-profile collapses of two other would-be pioneers: the Coquihalla highway project and the Vancouver Conventional Centre expansion.

The Coquihalla P3, announced in February 2002, was slated to be a fifty-five-year DBFO with tolls imposed for the first thirty-five years, but it was quickly abandoned in light of concerted public objection to the private tolling scheme in particular. Once tolls became politically impossible, the revenue streams needed to attract private investment also dried up and the DBFO model was scrapped. In 2003 the P3 was scaled down significantly, and it is now a much more limited operation-maintenance partnership, and no tolls were imposed on the highway. With respect to the Convention Centre expansion, negotiations collapsed in December 2002 when the preferred bidder pulled out as the result of a disagreement over revenue sharing and risk transfer. This was partially related to public outcry that centred on the proposal to establish a casino on the premises in order to generate the revenue needed to attract private investors.

These early Liberal-era collapsed deals provided important lessons for P3 policy design. First, public resistance to P3s could and would lead to significant results – even to an outright rejection of the model, highlighting the importance of depoliticization as a long-run goal for proponents. Furthermore, since these high-profile collapses occurred prior to the establishment of the provincial enabling field, it did little in the long run to squash subsequent P3 prominence. Second, the need to ensure that P3s offer private investors adequate and guaranteed returns on investment was demonstrated through both collapsed deals. This narrowed the range of potential P3 projects but bolstered the commitment to those that were feasible. The Canadian health care sector is thus "ideal" for privatization by stealth, given that the government is the purchaser of P3 infrastructure and services, not the public (i.e., patients), avoiding the need for user fees and guaranteeing strong and predictable rates of return for investors. Profitability for the Diamond Centre's private partner has also been boosted by the commercialization of hospital space, a feature unique to this hospital in its regional health authority. Thus early Liberal-era collapsed deals did not discourage BC's P3 enthusiasm; rather, they provided important lessons. Ultimately, the Coquihalla and Convention Centre projects were the only provincial-level P3 pioneers that did not come to fruition.[2]

History

Built in the early 1950s, the Matsqui-Sumas-Abbotsford (MSA) hospital was run down by the late 1980s and functionally obsolete by the end of the 1990s, not even capable of powering up the high-tech equipment that had become standard in most other hospitals. Beginning in the early 1980s, a

---

2 The Seymour Water Filtration Plant is another prime example of an early Liberal-era collapsed P3 deal; however, this was a municipal project and not a provincial-level initiative.

replacement hospital had been proposed by local health authorities. Recognizing this need, the NDP government had made promises over the course of its tenure to replace the hospital, but these were never fulfilled. Then, mere months before the 2001 election, the Abbotsford Hospital and Cancer Centre was announced and appeared in the 2001 NDP budget, to be publicly financed, built, and operated. The hospital again appeared in the spring 2002 Liberal budget as a public project, but by late 2001 the government had hired the accounting firm PricewaterhouseCoopers to provide an assessment of the private-for profit options available to deliver this facility. By November 2002 the PricewaterhouseCoopers evaluation was complete, and premier Gordon Campbell stated for the first time, in a speech made to the Independent Contractors and Builders Association of BC, that the hospital would "go private" (Dix 2003). In their spring 2003 Budget, the hospital was dropped from the government's capital plans as they sought to take advantage of accounting rules that at the time favoured P3s through off-book financing – allowing P3s to appear as lease payments in the provincial budget rather than upfront capital costs as with traditional infrastructure procurement.

Addressing very different needs, the process of redeveloping the Vancouver General Hospital's (VGH) teaching and ambulatory outpatient care facilities[3] would soon be forever twinned with the Abbotsford greenfield hospital project, since they were the first P3 hospitals in the province and developed at roughly the same time. Financial planning for the VGH Diamond Centre began in late 2001, and by early 2002 the health authority's proposal had been targeted by government as a potential P3 (BC Select Standing Committee on Public Accounts 2011). In October 2002 Premier Campbell announced that the redevelopment of VGH offices and teaching facilities would be BC's first P3 hospital project (also making it Canada's first DBFO hospital). Without the province having developed or evaluated a single P3 hospital, Premier Campbell promised that this P3 would be the "first of many" (Middleton 2002).

Justifying and Initiating P3 Use

By nearly all accounts the new hospital in Abbotsford is of high-quality design. It has garnered many accolades, including for its use of natural

---

3 "Ambulatory care" refers to specialty outpatient clinics, diagnostic and testing facilities, and physicians' offices.

light and other green features, its top-of-the-line infection-control design, and its spacious and time-saving layout (e.g., wards are oriented around a central hub) (Lewis 2008). It is also three times the size of the hospital that it replaced, has nearly 100 additional beds, a much larger emergency room, and allowed for high-tech care and cancer care to be provided for the first time in the region (ibid.). Yet aside from the obvious benefits that a new hospital and well-designed facility have provided for patients and staff, why exactly privatization (particularly a long-term bundled P3 agreement) was necessary remains an unanswered question. The government's explanation for this decision has varied over the years, owing more to scandal and public pressure than to forthrightness and transparency.

The initial explanation provided by government was that a P3 would offer cost savings, with the PricewaterhouseCoopers evaluation being used to support claims of P3 superiority. This rationale soon evaporated when a technological glitch revealed the redacted portions of the study, details that public service advocates and health care unions had been fighting for some time to access. When the specifics of the study were revealed, they raised serious concerns. PricewaterhouseCoopers concluded that a P3 could at best deliver a cost savings of 1 per cent, and this was if all went smoothly; it could deliver a savings of 5 per cent if some clinical services were privatized, in violation of the Canada Health Act (Sandler 2002; Cohn 2008, 77). After examining the report, forensic accountant Ron Parks proclaimed that it "relie[d] on 'suspect data,' [was] inconclusive and 'should not be used as the basis for a definitive government decision'" ("Private Hospital Schemes" 2002). This effectively eliminated the cost-savings argument.

Running concurrent to these developments were the ideological justifications being offered in 2001 and 2002. Here too the government held steadfast in the face of opposition, which in this case extended beyond unions and advocacy groups as province-wide public opinion polls were clearly indicating significant, widespread opposition to private involvement in the development of the new Abbotsford hospital (e.g., "Private Hospital in Abbotsford" 2002). Aside from the general P3-friendly atmosphere that began with the Liberal election victory in 2001, more specific evidence of an ideological bias first emerged a few months after the election when a memo sent by the Ministry of Health Services and Health Planning to each regional health authority informed them that the ministry would soon be "set[ting] criteria around which patient populations would be best served in a private setting" (Harrison 2001). Thus the desire to introduce privatization and marketization began in earnest.

By mid-2002 Premier Campbell stated to journalists, shortly after creating Partnerships BC and implementing the Capital Asset Management Framework (CAMF), "One of the things I think we have to do is *we have to be committed* to trying to getting the ones [P3s] that work out there" (Enchin 2002, emphasis added). A few months later, in November 2002, the Abbotsford hospital P3 was announced and finance minister Gary Collins is quoted as saying, "The project was not only important as an individual health facility but also *for the future of the P3 model in British Columbia*" (Goldsworthy 2002, emphasis added). From this Cohn (2008, 77) concludes, "Some projects had to be first, and the Abbotsford Hospital was seen as a good candidate," since the Abbotsford region was a strong Liberal support base and this reduced the political risks involved.

In order to see this "pilot project" come to fruition, commitment to the P3 model meant not only creating the initial contours of an enabling field and pushing forward with flimsy cost-savings arguments and thinly veiled ideological ambitions, but also disciplining local public health authorities who questioned the suitability of a P3 for their proposed facility. Mike Marasco, chief project officer for the Fraser Health Authority (FHA), was an outspoken champion of the P3 route but other members of this regional health authority (RHA) were less convinced (many of whom had extensive private sector finance and real estate experience). When they expressed scepticism about the use of a DBFO P3 early on in the process, the provincial government ordered the Board of Directors to accept the project as a P3 or face removal (Cohn 2008).[4] The RHA had instead preferred a less involved design-build P3 on the grounds that the project was too small to generate sufficient competition (and thus capture the gains promised) and that traditional financing and operations arrangements would be preferable (ibid.). Having

---

4 A similar incident also occurred with the FHA with respect to the Surrey Ambulatory Care Facility. Through a freedom-of-information request by the BC Health Coalition, it was revealed that during a meeting with the deputy health minister in 2006, the chair of the FHA, Keith Purchase, stated in relation to the Surrey facility, "P3s are the not the first choice of the committee" (reported in Sandborn 2007). At a separate committee meeting Purchase elaborates, "If we undertake the traditional partnerships strategy (P3) there is a lesser ability to control design, longer lead times and additional risk" (ibid.). A P3 was later chosen to develop this project. Keith Purchase resigned as chair of the FHA in 2007, stating that his departure was due partially to the demands placed on the FHA by the provincial government to follow "a budget process which compelled me to keep my board colleagues out of the loop" (ibid.).

lost confidence in the RHA to shepherd the nascent P3, several staff members were shuffled into other positions, and a special-purpose operating company was created to interface with the private consortia on behalf of the public partner. Guided by Partnerships BC and headed by Marasco (as chief project officer of the FHA), the operating company was intentionally designed to be at arm's length from the RHA (ibid.). The opaque nature of this arrangement also ensured that stakeholders were effectively kept in dark about the scope of the Abbotsford P3. Up until spring 2008 – just sixty days prior to the hospital's opening – the Hospital Employees' Union (HEU) knew only that the infrastructure would be a P3, and they were not told that the project agreement would include the full range of non-clinical support services (e.g., dietary services, housekeeping, maintenance, etc.) (R. Knox, director, membership services, HEU, interview, 29 November 2012).

Established in 2003 and named Abbotsford Hospital and Cancer Centre Inc. (AHCC), this operating company acts as the public partner in the P3 arrangement. It has representatives from the Ministry of Health, Partnerships BC (and the chairman of AHCC is also the former head of Partnerships BC), the relevant health authorities (FHA and, because of the cancer care component, the Provincial Health Services Authority), and the Fraser Valley Regional Hospital District. Despite this combined expertise, value for money claims have since been exposed as being suspect at best, to be examined shortly.

Like the Abbotsford hospital, the Diamond Centre renovation and expansion was clearly needed, and the building now houses forty offices that had previously been scattered around the VGH area. The improved layout has earned the facility an 84 per cent satisfaction rate by the patients who use it (BC Select Standing Committee on Public Accounts 2011). On the other hand, there are also limits to this type of satisfaction-based assessment given that, as the auditor general reports, external stakeholders such as taxpayers and other government agencies do not have an adequate way to rate their satisfaction with the new facility (Auditor General 2011, 12).

One negative aspect of the design is its single heating and cooling system. The project agreement assigns responsibility for heating and cooling to the private partner from 7 a.m. to 7 p.m. Within this ambulatory care facility, doctors' offices close at 5 p.m. Should the public partner wish to have the building open before/after that time, heating and cooling becomes their responsibility. The restrictive nature of these hours meant that the services provided by the sterile processing department had to coincide mainly with when doctors' offices were open, an inefficient and ineffective arrangement; and if sterile processing was to be done after 7 p.m., the public partner would have to pay for heating and cooling throughout the entire building, given the single HVAC system. The latter would be far too costly for the health authority, and thus it determined that the sterile processing department would require separate heating and cooling. Arranging for the private partner to alter the HVAC system on one floor alone cost the RHA roughly $55,000, as well as a 15 per cent administration fee (public partner manager 1, interview, 29 October 2012). This stands as an important indicator of several problematic elements of P3 agreements: the additional (hidden) costs for the public sector and the inherently inflexible nature of these agreements. Given that HVAC repairs could be done only through the private partner, this was not necessarily the most cost-effective scenario.

The Diamond Centre facility, as with the Abbotsford example, lacks a solid justification for being developed as a P3. In October 2002 it was announced that the Vancouver Coastal Health Authority (VCHA) would begin searching for a private partner, but value for money had yet to be established and the official report was released only two years later, in November 2004. As one reporter commenting on the 2002 announcement put it at the time, "Premier Gordon Campbell's plan to use a private-public partnership to build a new wing at the Vancouver General Hospital may sound good to him, but he has to let the rest of B.C. in on why" ("Campbell Dodged Questions" 2002). This sentiment was echoed by other news reports, which stated that there was no clear explanation ever given for how the P3 could save money in the long run (e.g., Middleton 2002).

Unlike the relatively high-profile development of the Abbotsford hospital, the establishment of the Diamond Centre P3 flew under the radar, arousing far less public attention. There are several likely reasons for this. First, it is due, at least partially, to the nature of the project itself. Since the Diamond Centre P3 involved mainly redesigning clinics and offices and was less than a third of the cost of the Abbotsford greenfield project, the latter was the more obvious cause for public concern at the time. Second, the Diamond Centre did not receive as much attention from public sector unions. With both pioneering P3s being developed at roughly the same time, the smaller size and scope of the Diamond Centre project made it a relatively less important target than the Abbotsford project, which was set to affect hundreds of support-service workers for decades to come.

A related explanation for the low profile of the Diamond Centre P3 pertains to the labour-relations climate at the time. Public sector unions such as the HEU (BC's health care services division of the Canadian Union of Public Employees) have been, and remain, a strong source of resistance against P3s. Yet at the time that the Diamond Centre was being developed, the HEU was also facing significant assault imposed by Bill 29-2002 (The Health and Social Services Delivery Improvement Act) and later Bill 37-2004 (The Health Sector [Facilities Subsector] Collective Agreement Act).

Bill 29-2002 was introduced shortly after the Liberal victory and allowed for the elimination or alteration of several key provisions in signed collective agreements, namely those that provided job security and protection from privatization. This new legislation applied to all "non-clinical" employees in BC's health sector. Within a few short years, more than 9,000 members of the HEU had lost their jobs, and wages were slashed and benefits cut in newly contracted-out positions (Cohen and Cohen 2006). In the Abbotsford region, contracting-out first took place in 2004 at the older Matsqui-Sumas-Abbotsford hospital, affecting all HEU housekeeping staff (i.e., prior to when the P3 opened in 2008). Many of the support-service contracts had been awarded to Sodexo, the company that later came to form the service partner of the winning private consortia (along with Johnson Controls). Thus Bill 29-2002 brought the threat of privatization to staff working in *all* hospitals, not only those subject to P3 arrangements. Further, Bill 37-2004 imposed wage rollbacks affecting 43,000 hospital and long-term health care workers and allowed for greater casualization of health sector employment (HEU 2004b). In light of wider concerns at the time, it is no surprise that the Diamond Centre P3 received little attention.

Finally, the low visibility of the Diamond Centre deal can be attributed to the enthusiasm and leadership displayed by the RHA. Unlike with the Abbotsford P3 planning process, the Diamond Centre project began as a business case initiated by VCHA. The RHA also led the planning and procurement stages of development (with input from the University of British Columbia's Faculty of Medicine), and the Ministry of Health and Partnerships BC acted only as process observers during these phases (Auditor General 2011). After the winning consortium was selected, negotiations with the private partner were headed up by VCHA. Once the negotiations with the preferred partner were nearly complete, in April 2004 the private accountancy firm Ernst & Young was contracted by the RHA to review the financial modelling (CPP

AACC 2004, 4); and Partnerships BC was contracted by VCHA to assist with writing the value for money report after the project agreement was in place (BC Select Standing Committee on Public Accounts 2011).

Thus from the start the Diamond Centre was relatively depoliticized when compared with the Abbotsford hospital. However, flying under the radar came at the expense of the routinization and institutionalization enjoyed by the latter, since it was the VCHA that led the entire process, not a team of experts and wider variety of stakeholders like we see with AHCC. This meant that a local health authority with no prior knowledge of P3 procedures was responsible for selecting the preferred private partner and negotiating with a multinational private consortium. When pressed for details about the negotiations in 2004, VCHA spokesperson Viviana Zanocco refused to name the preferred partner with whom discussions had already begun, and was surprisingly candid when she said, "In terms of timelines or deadlines or anything like that ... it's the first time we've done it, so we have no way of knowing how long it's supposed to take" (O'Connor 2004).

More significantly, this lack of routines and expertise foreshadowed the misleading nature of value for money claims. In 2011 BC's auditor general found that the "VCHA did not have a clear understanding of the scope and user requirements before going to market for a private partner," and a number of undesirable outcomes were the result (2011a, 11). They included changes to the functional design of the facility *after* the project agreement had been signed, meaning the changes were paid for entirely by the VCHA, even though in 2004 scope risks were said to have been transferred to the private partner (Partnerships BC 2004). Altogether, the lack of expertise amounted to variations that cost the RHA $10.68 million (Auditor General 2011, 11). CAMF protocols now ensure that the functional design is complete before the P3 route is initiated. Another major bungle appeared in the recordkeeping procedures of the VCHA, as the BC auditor general found that by 2011 there was no longer any documentation available to support the 2004 value for money report released to the public.

Value for Money?

Both official value for money reports produced by Partnerships BC claim that these two P3s were delivered "on time" and "on budget" (Partnerships BC 2004; 2005). Yet arriving at this determination requires adopting an extremely narrow interpretation of these terms, with the Abbotsford P3 construction costs increased by 68 per cent, from an estimated $211 million in 2001 when the project was first announced, to $355 million in 2004 when construction actually began (Palmer 2008). This cost increase is due partially to changes (improvements) in design, yet can also be traced back to the lengthy contract negotiations inherent with complex P3 arrangements. These protracted negotiations pushed the initiation of the project into a booming construction market and added $63 million in inflation costs alone (Cayo 2005). It also delayed the opening of the hospital. Originally, in 2003, British Columbians were told that the P3 route would mean faster delivery – that construction would begin in 2004 and the hospital would open in early 2007 (Harrison 2003) – but bidding and contract negotiation delayed the project by nearly two years and the hospital began accepting patients only in late 2008. This is not reflected in Partnerships BC's (2005) official value for money report, and instead the hospital is labelled as being on time and on budget, since once the agreement was in place, the hospital was delivered as specified.

The Diamond Centre track record fares slightly better, although it too was late and more costly than originally promised. In 2002 the Campbell Liberals touted the P3 model as a way of delivering the facility by spring 2005, at a cost of $90 million (O'Connor 2004), yet it ended up opening in fall 2006 at a purported cost of $95 million (Partnerships BC 2004). However, as it turns out, discussed in greater detail below, there is no basis of support for this figure of $95, million and instead the final capitalized value of the redevelopment project is $123 million (Auditor General 2011, 9). There are also the additional (hidden) costs associated with very minor items that should not be overlooked. Hanging a picture in an office, for example, is not only a "hassle" for the health authority, since it has to be arranged through the private partner (i.e., VCHA cannot use their own maintenance staff), but it also may be more costly since VCHA cannot use the cheapest vendor, and the private partner charges a 15 per cent overhead fee each time a service such as this is provided (public partner manager 1, interview, 29 October 2012).

Perhaps of greater concern than the delays and cost creep is that value for money has never been clearly established with either hospital, despite adamant claims of P3 superiority by Partnerships BC. The P3 route was chosen well before value for money had been adequately assessed, even though best practice (now and at the time) dictated that it be established in advance, since this is supposed to be the basis upon which the selection of a P3 is made.

The methodology used to later produce the value for money assessments was also angled in favour of privatization. With the Abbotsford P3 a discount rate of 6 per cent was used to determine value for money, when in the United Kingdom (pioneers of the P3) best practice dictates using a rate of 3.5 per cent (Parks and Terhart 2009, 8). At a rate of 6 per cent, delivering the hospital as a P3 appeared to save $39 million, but this result is highly sensitive. Forensic accountants Parks and Terhart calculate that at 4.5 per cent neither the P3 nor the PSC is favoured, and at a rate of 3.5 per cent a publicly delivered hospital would produce a savings of roughly $80 million when compared to the P3 option. On this basis, Parks and Terhart conclude that the methodology used to determine value for money in the Abbotsford case was "biased in favour of the P3" (16).

Erroneous value for money claims are similarly present in the official value for money report produced by Partnerships BC for the Diamond Centre. The report claims that the leading factors supporting a P3 were that the project would offer a good return on private investment, that a P3 would be the most cost-effective option from a life-cycle cost perspective, and that a P3 would offer other benefits such as risk transfer, timely delivery, and innovation (Partnerships BC 2004, 4). Yet in his 2011 assessment, BC's auditor general found that many of these promises did not materialize, with the important exception of offering a good return on private investment. For instance, variations in the functional design led the auditor to conclude, "The P3 agreement in this case did not effectively manage the project scope risk" (Auditor General 2011, 11). The value for money report also suggests that the RHA's operational risks are minimized, given that payments made to the private operator and service-provider can be adjusted on the basis of performance (Partnerships BC 2004). However, the auditor's report reveals that "the quantitative performance standards set out in the Service Requirements were not measured and monitored" (12). Without any effective ability to measure and monitor performance, this risk is certainly not transferred.

Financial savings are also highlighted in the Diamond Centre's official value for money report, with it claiming that the P3 option would save $17 million in net present value terms compared to the PSC (Partnerships BC 2004). These calculations used a discount rate of 7.12 per cent on the grounds that this rate "reflected the inherent risks transferred to the private partner" (11). BC's auditor general would later conclude that this discount rate was too high and ought to have been more accurately set at 5.37 per cent. Using the lower and more appropriate rate adds $17 million to the total capitalized value of the P3 project (Auditor General 2011, 6). This adjustment, along with the nearly $11 million cost increase due to the functional design variations discussed above, means that the final capitalized value of the P3 was actually $123 million – which amounts to $28 million above the 2004 figure (see Auditor General 2011). Scope changes aside, this final value is well in excess of the PSC generated at the time.

High transaction costs are also present with these P3 hospitals. With the Abbotsford hospital, the BC provincial government spent over $7 million in administrative costs, and $24.7 million on legal and consultant costs (Partnerships BC 2005, 34). Given that the Diamond Centre was developed by the VCHA, it had to hire private advisors to the tune of $2.4 million, or 2.5 per cent of the project's total estimated capital costs in 2004 (Partnerships BC 2004, 7).

All told, the delays, increased costs, poor value for money, high transaction costs, and methodological biases greatly undermine any financial/economic rationale upon which these P3s could be justified. Satisfactory architectural design and functionality of these projects hardly outweigh all of the drawbacks. Politically, we see that the strong ideological desire to have P3 hospitals developed in the province led to broken promises by government officials and little transparency overall. Despite this strong political support at all levels of government, there is also no accountability assumed by P3 proponents. The bad choices, poor results, and ongoing concerns have been neither acknowledged nor addressed.

Private Partners, Private Services

With the Abbotsford hospital, the private partner holds a thirty-year lease on the facility and was awarded responsibility for design, construction, finance, maintenance, and management and operation of the hospital (involving general management, help desk, food services for patients and non-patients, housekeeping, laundry and linen services, material services, plant services including facility maintenance, protection services, patient portering, utilities management, and parking services) (Partnerships BC 2005, 17). In-house management of patient portering for oncology services was retained by the BC Cancer Agency (R. Knox, interview, 29 November 2012). In the case of the Diamond Centre, the private partner also holds a thirty-year lease and was similarly awarded responsibility for design, construction, finance, maintenance, and management and operation (involving housekeeping, security, groundskeeping, and leasing space not used by the public partner) (Partnerships BC 2004, 9–12). These "full spectrum" P3s (or DBFOs) are the norm for BC hospital partnerships, although there are some variations. For instance, the Interior

Health Authority has exempted some cleaning services from its P3 deals, but all other support services are included. Elsewhere in the province, P3 hospital deals include "hard" facility services such as maintenance, help desk, and physical plant, but "soft" services tend to be limited to house-keeping (for an up-to-date list, see Partnerships BC n.d.).

Both hospitals' winning private partner consortia were composed of large, mainly multinational actors. For Access Health Abbotsford (AHA), financing was provided and arranged by ABN AMRO Bank, facilities management and support services are operated by Johnson Controls and Sodexo, and construction was handled by PCL Construc-tors. Similarly, Access Health Vancouver (AHV) involved financing from ABN AMRO, PCL oversaw the construction, and Johnson Con-trols now manages the facility. Architectural design was provided by different private partners: Silver Thomas Hanley and Musson Cattell Mackey (AHA) and IBI/HPA (AHV). Thus the Abbotsford private partner was composed of only two Canadian firms (PCL and Musson Cattell Mackey), as was the Diamond Centre (PCL and IBI/HPA).

The composition of the private partner subsequently changed for both P3 hospitals. Originally financed by the Dutch bank ABN AMRO, in 2005 it sold its share in each partnership to the Australian investment bank Macquarie; and in 2007 this was sold once more to John Laing PLC. These P3 hospitals therefore had three different owners in as many years (2005–7) (CUPE 2011, 11; Sandborn 2008). Refinancing is a huge source of profits for private P3 partners (see Whitfield 2009), and John Laing PLC, the current financial partner for both P3 hospitals, was criticized in 2008 by the chair of the U.K. House Public Accounts Committee for rep-resenting "the unacceptable face of capitalism" for its 2003 refinancing of a U.K. PFI hospital which led to "windfall" profits and a 60 per cent return on investment (Sandborn 2008). In BC, P3 hospital agreements contain clauses that require the private partner to share half of all rev-enue earned through refinancing with the public partner.

With the Diamond Centre, AHV won through competitive bidding, although, as noted above, selection was highly opaque. On the other hand, AHA won the contract when the other three potential bidders dropped out, confirming earlier fears expressed by the RHA surround-ing poor market competition. When there is only a single candidate, a primary argument in support of P3s is eliminated: that competition for the P3 contract will ultimately benefit taxpayers and service users. With only one bidder, best practice is often to move away from a DBFO by unbundling some of the project's components. AHCC member, and chief project officer for the FHA at the time, Mike Marasco defends their choice to go with AHA's bid: "We may have ended up with one at the very end, but we started with four strong teams, and thanks to the process that we've put in place, there was competitive pressure put on the final team in the homestretch because they had already spent a significant amount of money on preparing their bid ... we had an intensely competitive bid that resulted in our having an innovative design and a project that we could say we expect to receive value for money from" (BC Select Standing Committee on Public Accounts 2006). The private fairness auditor hired to evaluate this irregularity also concluded that it was a competitive process. Yet an initially competitive process is not necessarily the same as competitive market pressures producing the best value for money. Ultimately AHCC partnered with the only consortium that had not withdrawn their bid – hardly a ringing endorsement for the preferred proponent and the benefits of a P3.

P3 value for money analyses fare poorly in capturing the social concerns associated with the use of private for-profit service operators. Social costs can vary, but in the health care sector they typically relate to problems with inadequate training, poor hygiene control, and deep cuts made to wages and benefits (e.g., "BC Health Authorities" 2009; Cohen and Cohen 2006; Leyne 2009). In January 2004 many of the support services at the Matsqui-Sumas-Abbotsford hospital were contracted out to Sodexo – a multinational corporation specializing in food services and building maintenance in hospitals, schools, prisons, and similar institutions, with a record of industrial standards violations and union-busting (HEU 2004a) – and the very same company that would soon be a member of the private consortia awarded the Abbotsford P3 contract. Within four months (April 2004), the *Abbotsford Times* found evidence of declining standards in the hospital. For example, it reported on "tales of blood smears in labour rooms that should be spotless, litter left behind in beds in the emergency ward and inexperienced workers entering infectious isolation rooms" (quoted in HEU 2004a). Inadequate training may have contributed to this, with the HEU hearing that newly privatized staff were given only a day of training, outside of a hospital setting (R. Knox, interview, 29 November 2012).

There have yet to be any reports of this occurring at the P3 hospital, but in fall 2012 Sodexo's cleanliness and infection-control standards were once again in the news with the outbreak of the superbug *C. difficile* in Burnaby Hospital (like Abbotsford, this hospital is also in the FHA). The outbreak led the HEU to call for a housekeeping audit, given that Sodexo passed cleaning standards, despite the infectious outbreak. The union claims that "right now hospital cleaning is based on visual appearances only" (HEU 2012, 1). When housekeeping services are kept in-house rather than privatized, the public sector retains full control over the types of cleaning products used and method of cleaning, as well as the number of staff employed. Private partners, on the other hand, have a vested interest in getting work done quickly and at a low cost. With hospital staff often working in several different hospitals each day, the implications of cut corners in any one facility can easily reverberate across the whole region (R. Knox, interview, 29 November 2012).

Problems with the Diamond Centre's housekeeping subcontractor Bee-Clean have also emerged. According to one interviewee, "They [Bee-Clean] don't understand how to clean up a clinical unit" (public partner manager 1, interview, 29 October 2012). The performance of this cleaning subcontractor remains an "ongoing frustration" for the public partner and they "just aren't happy with the service" (ibid.; also stated by public partner manager 2, interview, 8 November 2012). Bee-Clean is a Canadian janitorial and building-maintenance company and does not specialize in health sector housekeeping. Despite the dissatisfaction of the health authority, the P3 project agreement awards full control over housekeeping services to the private partner (AHV). Thus AHV, not VCHA, chooses the subcontractor for these services.

The Abbotsford project agreement, on the other hand, is more robust in its support-service provisions. The project agreement allows for "market testing" every five years (meaning that a service-provider's overall performance is graded at regular intervals), and this applies to all privatized services except for general management (i.e., AHA itself) and physical plant, which is considered a life-cycle risk, where performance (and risk transfer) can be truly established only at the end of the thirty-year project agreement. The first five-year period for market testing is 2008–13. The review began in summer 2012 (looking at scores, surveys, other performance indicators), and if the expectations set out in the project agreement were met, the price paid by the RHA for the private partner's services was to remain the same – and hence subcontractors would likely be retained. The incentive for good performance is therefore instilled principally within subcontractors. The private partner is able to pass on any payment deductions that it faces to the vendors it has hired, raising the question of what risk AHA truly holds during the operational phase of the project. By fall 2012 it appeared likely that, as the result of suboptimal performance, ten of twelve services provided by AHA would be "taken back to market" in 2013. In other words, ten of twelve subcontractors have been performing below expectations.

Low wages and benefits are another feature of BC's privatized health care support services. As mentioned, in 2002 Bill 29 rescinded signed collective agreements, cutting wages for staff now employed by the province's "Big Three" private contractors (Sodexo, Aramark, and Compass Group) nearly in half, to $9–$10 per hour, and rolling back benefits. By 2004–7 the HEU had organized most contracted-out support staff in the province. The first round of bargaining began in 2004 and this led to a $3–$4/hour wage increase (HEU 2008). The next round of bargaining began in 2008 and produced a 15 per cent wage gain ($15 per hour by 2011). These improvements are significant and the HEU has acknowledged Sodexo's willingness to work with the union; however, the effects of Bill 29 are still being felt a decade after its implementation, given that nominal hourly wages in 2012 were in many instances below what they were in 2002. In contrast, P3 agreements like the one governing the Abbotsford hospital provide for yearly inflation-adjusted increases in service payments made to private contractors. Furthermore, privatization is now clearly entrenched within the public health care system. Regional health authorities no longer employ the vast majority of support staff in BC's health sector, although the opposite was true in 2001.

The internal bifurcation of authority within the Abbotsford hospital has also meant that staff cannot hang pictures without the private owners' approval, or even signs addressing workplace safety concerns. In some instances bifurcation may be little more than an annoyance; in others it hinders service delivery. Given the "true employer" provisions of Bill 94-2003 and 29-2002, work directions for privatized staff can come only from private managers. Thus public and private hospital staff are effectively "kept segregated," even when such an arrangement disrupts the timeliness of cleaning services (R. Knox, interview, 29 November 2012).

Operations, Contracting Monitoring, and Enforcement

The Diamond Centre contains an element of commercialization: commercial and retail activities have been incorporated into the project agreement in order to allow for greater profitability. Provisions for rental revenue stipulate that the private partner, AHV, is able to keep all profit up to a certain threshold, above which a percentage is shared with the health authority (CPP AACC 2004). In exchange, AHV holds the risk that this space may be vacant. Because it is located within a large hospital and health services area, as well as a prime retail location within the city of Vancouver itself, this risk has not yet materialized. The retail space has been consistently occupied by eateries, coffee shops, and since 2006 the large pharmacy chain Shoppers Drug Mart. There are currently no other examples of for-profit commercial retail space in VCHA hospitals (public partner manager 1, interview, 29 October 2012). Small gift shops are a feature common to traditional hospitals, but these are run by charitable organizations and hospital auxiliaries with revenue dedicated to patient services/support. An exception is the retail coffee shop Café Ami run by Sodexo in the Jim Pattison Outpatient Care and Surgical Centre; however, this is also a P3 facility and Sodexo holds the food services contract.

Although comparative data are lacking, it would be fair to say that for most privatized hospital staff, P3 environments can be nearly identical to contracting-out. However, for public sector authorities the operational phase of the P3 agreement presents particular challenges that set the two forms of privatization apart. First, P3 agreements are far longer, and second, all contracts are bundled into one agreement. Thus a P3 private partner does not face the discipline that accompanies contracting-out, since those contracts are renewed every few years, not every few decades. Further, the private partners of a P3 enjoy a monopoly, given that even in the case of very poor performance it is not legally possible to sever any one portion of a project agreement without renegotiating the entire project agreement – which in most instances would be a prohibitively expensive, time-consuming ordeal.

The long-term and bundled nature of P3 contracts also means that most components contributing to value for money, risk transfer, and cost savings – the foundational justifications of the P3 model – ultimately manifest during the operational phase of any given project. Contract monitoring and the enforcement of performance standards are therefore integral to reaping the purported rewards of a P3. Yet the Diamond Centre agreement does not actually allow the public partner to alter service payments in the case of poor performance or service non-availability (Auditor General 2011). Should problems arise with housekeeping and security services, for example, there are provisions in the agreement that allow the private partner to release subcontractors, but there is no such power given to the public partner to impose payment deductions. Dealing with these issues from the public partner's perspective thus requires "developing a long-term relationship and working together" (public partner manager 2, interview, 8 November 2012). This stands in stark contrast to the typical P3 proponent rhetoric of using private contracts to insulate the public from unnecessary cost and risk.

For the Abbotsford hospital there is a different concern about risk transfer (or the lack thereof) during the operational phase of the P3 – it appears to be common practice for the provisions in the project agreement to be overlooked, and, in at least one instance, changed for the benefit of the private partner. Statements made at a private seminar by the general manager of AHCC, the Abbotsford P3 public partner, are especially revealing (public partner manager 3, private seminar, 31 October 2012):

> I don't ever check that project agreement, I only check the writing in the book as a very last [step] ... I figure out what the right thing is to do and I sit down with the private people and say, "Here's the right thing," and we reach agreement and then we go back and make the language of the book fit what the right thing is.
>
> I haven't gone to dispute, haven't gone to the lawyers in the [several] years that I've been there, because I've been able to find the happy medium, the win-win.
>
> We had a payment deduction that we were entitled to millions of dollars from our private partners, and my belief and the belief of my board was that it was too strong a payment deduction for them. It would have bankrupted them and they would have gone out of business. It was just an error in the writing of the project agreement. It was way too severe a penalty for something so minor, so we actually settled on something substantially less than that because it was the right thing to do, and then we corrected the book. We actually went back into the book, did an appendix to the project agreement.

While there can be no doubt that managing a complex, thirty-year relationship requires compromise on all sides, it is unlikely that a private partner would be willing to return these favours. In fact, a public partner manager (ibid.) further stated, with respect to the millions of dollars owed to AHCC for a particular payment deduction, "They [AHV] believed that they didn't have to pay us [AHCC] anything." Not only do these day-to-day practices defy the "market-discipline" and "risk transfer" promises of those promoting P3s, but they also reveal the deep reorientation of public sector decision-making: public hospital managers now thoroughly incorporate and accommodate the interests of private for-profit partners.

Proliferation

BC's pioneering P3 hospitals clearly suffer from several major problems: cost creep and delays lead to broken promises with little public accountability or recognition that this has occurred; P3 development proceeds without having been subject to a proper value for money analysis; value for money assessments that are later produced use methodological techniques to justify the use of a P3 ex post facto; there are problems with bidding (Abbotsford) and changes made after the project agreement is in place (Diamond); dubious risk transfer; and both private partners composed of nearly the identical group of multinational corporations. At least some of these issues resulted from a lack of public sector expertise and were corrected through the routinization of P3 procurement and enabling field reforms. The next round of P3 hospitals were initiated several years later – the bulk of which were launched after 2007, some five years after Partnerships BC was up and running and the CAMF had been put in place. So the pertinent question becomes whether the problems exhibited by these pioneering P3s were isolated incidents due mainly to inexperience. In other words, what benefits, if any, have enabling fields provided? A full reporting of the similarities and differences would require a thorough examination of each new case; nevertheless several trends can be identified and listed here, leading to the conclusion that benefits have been procedural rather than substantial.

First, government ministries and the Office of the Premier in particular are no longer as directly involved, or at least they do not appear to be. The commitment to P3s has been maintained, and in fact expanded upon, as the number of P3 hospitals swells, but it now occurs in a far more depoliticized fashion. Depoliticization takes the two forms discussed in the previous chapter. Most obviously, decision-making is shifted from the public sector to the private sector as the number of P3 hospitals grows (the effects of which have yet to be fully seen, since only a small number are currently operational). Further, and likely of greater importance for the normalization of P3 policy, decision-making has been shifted from the governmental sphere to the realm of public and quasi-public authority. Partnerships BC has taken the lead role in determining the contours of negotiations, contract development, the selection of preferred bidders, in promoting privatization, and in guiding the regional health authorities with which it partners to represent the public interest. This is not to say that the Ministry of Health no longer participates in the P3 planning process, but its role is confined mainly to oversight tasks, such as approving the business case and sitting on the board of major capital projects. As with the Abbotsford example, the project board of all new major hospital capital projects is composed of representatives from the Ministry of Health, the Ministry of Transportation and Infrastructure, Partnerships BC, and the relevant regional health authority. The Ministry of Finance has maintained a strong indirect role through its CAMF. The creation of enabling field routines has meant that all P3 hospitals now follow the same series of steps to establish project scope, schedule, cost, and risks upfront rather than after the fact.

Along with procedural similarities comes a second trend, this one being of greater significance than is the streamlining and predictability identified above. Process harmonization without substantial evaluation of the appropriateness of the P3 model has meant that the accounting and methodological issues associated with the Abbotsford hospital and Diamond Centre P3 deals have not been ameliorated but instead systematically engrained and obscured through sophisticated technocratic techniques and routines.

Speaking to the Select Standing Committee on Public Accounts in 2011, Duncan Campbell, CFO of the VCHA, claimed that many lessons had been learned and processes improved upon since the Diamond Centre P3 was developed. For instance, he argued that "the accounting treatment is very clear now" and that "the rules have changed. They're much more transparent" (BC Select Standing Committee on Public Accounts 2011). This sentiment is echoed by representatives of Partnerships BC. In 2006, CEO Larry Blain also told a Select Standing Committee on Public Accounts, "The idea of producing a value for money report was an initiative of Partnerships B.C. Our intent was to raise the level of disclosure around major capital projects, and I believe that we are reporting out at a level of disclosure which is unprecedented in Canada" (BC Select Standing Committee on Public Accounts 2006).

These claims are misleading. Even though value for money reports are now conducted by Partnerships BC ahead of time and are displayed on their website – both of which were much-needed improvements – the amount of data that is actually made public leaves much to be desired. As John Loxley (2012, 22) put it, it is "impossible to deconstruct or reproduce VfM assessments," with the result that "transparency is really quite opaque, a form of window-dressing." The reason consistently offered by Partnerships BC is that this is needed to protect commercial confidentiality. While there may be some merit to this argument, it is also true that there is now an illusion of enhanced public disclosure and transparency but nearly the same level secrecy as in the past. Greater public access to some project details therefore goes a long way towards normalizing and depoliticizing P3s while doing very little to substantially improve outcomes and address concerns that P3s are anti-democratic.

Methodological issues also remain (Loxley 2012). Discount rates are still far too high, and thus value for money calculations remain mathematically biased against the PSC; risk transfer claims are still vague and lacking justification, though entirely relied upon as the basis for declaring P3 superiority; and oversight into these issues is still almost non-existent. When the auditor general reported on the Abbotsford hospital in 2006, it was merely an attestation report, not a direct audit. All that this exercise accomplished was to confirm that the numbers used by Partnerships BC did in fact add up; it did not independently verify any of the value for money data, and thus could not say where those numbers came from. When the Diamond Centre P3 was audited in 2011, the auditor general exposed many significant problems – but even this audit was limited. It did not tackle how and on what basis the P3 was developed (and thus whether a P3 should have been chosen at all), but instead assessed whether the project achieved three of its value for money goals, which it did not. By early 2015, the auditor general has yet to report on any other P3 hospital in the province. There is similar lack of official auditing for P3s in other sectors as well. Aside from the reports previously cited in this chapter, by January 2015 there was only one other P3-related report, concerning the Sea-to-Sky Highway Improvement Project and the Britannia Mine Water Treatment Plant Project (Auditor General 2012).

Another looming issue that has yet to fully reveal itself is the inadequate quantification of service outcomes, a concern also flagged by the auditor general (2011a) in his report on the Diamond Centre. Without adequate measurement, the public partner loses the ability to adjust the level of payments made to the private partner, and thus to control operational outcomes. Further, long-term monitoring and formal reporting on how operational P3s are functioning remain sorely lacking. All too often P3 policy champions point to, and focus resources on, the procurement and construction phases. In BC, public sector expertise targets the two or three years required to procure a deal – from Partnerships BC to the ministries involved (including the

Office of the Premier for pioneering P3s) as well as the private sector consultants and fairness monitors hired to ensure that value for money has been secured. Construction is another high-profile time for P3 hospitals, and proponents are quick to cite "on time" and "on budget" results. The operational phase of a P3 project, in contrast, unfolds over thirty years, and Partnerships BC has yet to put in place any systemic resources devoted to contract monitoring and operations management. As suggested by a public partner manager with AHCC (public partner manager 3, private seminar, 31 October 2012), "We only look at the sexy part of the business ... it's not hard to manage a budget when you can't go over time and over budget ... when you cut the ribbon, the purse strings are wide open, and you have to be really cognizant of what is happening in the operating thirty-year term ... I've been in this job for [several] years and I've probably had less than six hours of conversation with anyone [at Partnerships BC] asking me how it's going."

It is doubtful that greater transparency and contract management would significantly ameliorate the P3 model, but improvements in operational monitoring could help to ensure that the elements of cost savings and risk transfer that have been included in the project agreement are actually being achieved. It was only in 2011, nearly five years after the first P3 hospital opened its doors in BC, that Partnerships BC acknowledged that they needed to develop long-term monitoring and operational reporting procedures (BC Select Standing Committee on Public Accounts 2011). Some procedural changes have been made in light of the Diamond Centre service contract problems; for instance, contracts now "are much more specific" (ibid.), but the auditor general's (2011a) recommendations on operational management and improving the performance metrics have yet to be implemented by the VCHA.

Just as with the initiation of the P3 model in health care, there are few proactive protections for the public interest during the operational phase of these hospitals. Rather than anticipating the problems that might occur with P3s, it appears as though the BC provincial government and its agencies are satisfied simply to develop them without actually scrutinizing them.

The development of BC's P3 hospital market since its pioneering projects were launched also offers some cause for concern. It is a quirk of the Abbotsford and Diamond Centre agreements that both private partners were nearly identical, and this supported fears that concentration would occur and that smaller contractors and medium-sized companies in the province would be squeezed out (e.g., Knappett 2008). These concerns appear to paradoxically have been accurate and yet unfounded in the health sector. They are unfounded because smaller projects still go forward using either traditional or design-build P3 procurement, and private partners of large DBFOs subcontract their work to smaller local firms. There is also now a wider range of private partners bidding and winning than the AHV and AHA results would have suggested at the time (see Partnerships BC n.d.). On the other hand, these fears have also proven accurate, because within the DBFO P3 market it is still only the largest corporations (predominantly multinationals) that have been consistently awarded these contracts – and thus they control, and benefit the most from, large hospital (re)development projects in the province. Provisions prohibiting changes in private consortia membership, as occurred with the AHV and AHA financing partner, have yet to be implemented in BC. Changes in P3 ownership therefore remain beyond the control of government.

Concluding Remarks

The hospital P3s examined in this chapter provide important examples of the disconnect between the rhetoric of P3 proponents and the reality of P3 projects: the higher costs, lengthy bidding and negotiation stages, erroneous or misleading value for money claims, and social and labour concerns that arise from support service privatization. These projects also demonstrate the contradiction inherent in attempting to achieve value for money through *privatization*, given the realities of managing a decades-long *partnership*. Gaining the greatest possible number of public sector benefits from privatized P3 service-providers can come only from having a strong commitment to enforcing the project agreement, yet effective service provision requires the opposite: negotiation, compromise, and collaboration. The distinctive nature of the partnership aspect of a P3 has been affirmed by public and private partners alike (private partner manager 2, interview, 16 November 2012; public partner manager 1, interview, 29 October 2012; public partner manager 2, interview, 8 November 2012).

The ongoing proliferation of P3s in the face of problems and concerns lends support to Clarke's (2008) notion of neoliberal "doubling," or the way in which instances of neoliberalism are both integrated within and remake the whole (see also Peck 2010, 22). P3 pitfalls reflect problems inherent to the model yet simultaneously urge process (policy) change that suppresses or helps to ignore suboptimal outcomes. There is a model of P3 development that represents an ideal, the way these projects are "supposed to" work, and then there is the reality of how actual project development and operation functions. "Evidence" from each new project is marshalled by proponents to confirm the superiority of the P3 model, even when it is impossible to do so, given the rampant and uncorrected value for money errors and secrecy through commercial confidentiality; the pseudo-science that goes into these calculations; and the lack of any oversight and corrections made before new projects are initiated. Thus the "evidence" that is used to confirm the superiority of the model and justify future projects is based on circular reasoning and self-referentiality, and is intensely ideological, despite depoliticization.

It should also be pointed out that any discussion of P3 faults must be set within the context of earlier delays, broken promises, cost overruns, and low transparency with traditional projects. One of the strengths of the P3 model offered by industry proponents and scholarly analyses is that once project agreements are in place, the P3 contract ensures that the infrastructure will be built. However, this is less an argument in favour of P3s than it is a reminder that election promises are not always kept. Fixing public-procurement problems through public solutions was the obvious next step in BC, but this was never given the effort that establishing enabling fields and P3 projects received. There was, to reiterate, no obvious financial imperative urging on the P3 route with either facility. BC's initial P3 hospitals were pushed through by the government of the day on the basis of sheer political will, in the face of public opposition, protest by civil society groups, and concern expressed by members of the regional health authority (FHA), and with value for money having never been clearly established. Furthermore, tying the hands of future governments through binding multi-decade agreements can be equally interpreted as a negative aspect of P3s.

Given the propensity to increase the cost of infrastructure, as well as many other social disadvantages that accompany the use of P3s in health care, it is difficult to see how they create solutions to rising health sector costs today. The higher costs associated with P3 use not only undermine proponents' arguments that they help curb wasteful government spending, they also mean that less is available to be spent on future social concerns and other infrastructure projects. The legacy of broken promises, delays, higher costs, and hidden fees associated with P3s greatly undermines arguments that oppose traditional public infrastructure on the grounds that it is too costly for the cash-strapped provinces to afford.

Enabling fields may have marginally improved the P3 policy landscape today, but improvements have not reduced costs or increased public oversight and accountability – they have only made it appear as though this has happened. RID has made P3s more palatable, and thus more dangerous. This chapter has examined how that has happened in BC; next we look at how it has occurred in Ontario.

Chapter 6

Ontario's Pioneering P3 Hospitals

There is a complex relationship between the development of Ontario's initial P3 hospitals and the unfolding of its P3-enabling field. In contrast to the BC experience discussed in the previous chapter, P3 projects and policies did not emerge concurrently in Ontario, but instead the province's first DBFO hospitals were initiated by a different government and prior to the enabling field. First announced by the Mike Harris–led Progressive Conservative (PC) government in late 2001, the Brampton Civic Hospital and Royal Ottawa Hospital projects got off to a rocky start with much public resistance throughout the development process. Later, in the lead up to the October 2003 provincial election, these two P3s were again a hot topic and subject to much public, politicized debate. Concern over P3s would not be assuaged through abandonment of the model by the victorious Dalton McGuinty Liberals but instead through alterations (both rhetorical and real) to the hospital project agreements and the creation of a supportive edifice around P3 development – the provincial P3-enabling field. In so doing, the government shifted the policy emphasis from cost savings to efficiency, from necessity to prudence, from rollback to rollout. It is under these conditions that routinization, institutionalization, and depoliticization have allowed the P3 model to flourish in Ontario, and this province is now the single most important P3 market in the country. From a shaky start marred by years of delays and controversy, by 2012 there were over thirty P3s in development in Ontario's health sector.

This chapter examines the Brampton Civic Hospital and Royal Ottawa Hospital projects for their performance and legacy, including the historical and political circumstances under which they were created, value for money–related issues, operational concerns, and ways that subsequent P3 hospitals were affected by the legacy of the trailblazers. The appendix should also be consulted for its detail on the timeline and milestones of each P3.

Initiation: Ontario's Pioneering P3 Hospitals

Ontario's initial P3 hospitals were highly politicized, offered poor value for money, and came in much later and at a higher price than originally promised. This experience contributed to P3 policy alteration and the development of the current enabling field. A change in government in 2003 led to the amelioration of some concerning features of these project agreements, but it also opened the door to a much more systematic P3 program in the health sector. The new approach developed by the McGuinty Liberals was so successful that by 2008 the executive vice-president of Infrastructure Ontario estimated that roughly 75 per cent of all P3s in the province were hospitals (Ontario Standing Committee on Government Agencies 2008).

A common characteristic shared by the Brampton Civic Hospital and Royal Ottawa Hospital P3s is that, despite the decades-long need for these facilities, they suffered neglect under the traditional procurement model. This situation was not the result of an intrinsic failure of the public procurement model; funding was simply not made available, despite the clear need for each project. Perhaps because of this neglect the hospital boards responsible for these projects embraced either public or private involvement – whichever would prove most expedient. Yet regardless of any local "buy-in," the decision to use a P3 in both instances was never truly left up to the local authorities; it was a Cabinet-level initiative from the start and continued to be after the change in government in 2003. These projects indicate the features and failures of the earlier PC SuperBuild framework (a proto-enabling field) and illustrate the importance of the Liberal government's enabling field for the routinization, institutionalization, and depoliticization of the P3 health sector program.

Background

Ontario's use of P3s did not begin with the Dalton McGuinty Liberals in 2003 when the elements of the enabling field were first beginning to form or even with the PCs' Common Sense Revolution in 1995, but instead was touched off much earlier under the Bob Rae–led NDP government of the early 1990s. Prior to the Liberal victory, P3s were never a sector-wide affair, and only a handful had been developed in the province. "Experimentation" with this procurement model is the term that best captures P3 policy in the 1990s, as there was little effort made to systematize P3 use before Harris's second term, which started in 1999. This is not to say that individual P3 projects were insignificant, for several large, high-profile projects were developed in the 1990s in a range of sectors. For example, in the transportation sector there was the 1993 Highway 407 deal, and in social services there was the 1997 Ontario Business Transformation Project; municipally, in 1994 the Hamilton-Wentworth Water and Sewage System P3 agreement began. Each suffered several problems, from cut corners and safety concerns resulting from the profit motive (Highway 407), to collapsed deals and inadequate upkeep (Hamilton-Wentworth), to poor/unsubstantiated value for money (Business Transformation) (see Loxley 2010). Issues of this sort, combined with little effort to create an enabling field, kept P3 use relatively marginal throughout most of the 1990s.

In 1999 the situation began to change when the PC government was re-elected for a second term.[1] The Common Sense Revolution that ousted the NDP in 1995 was focused mainly on rolling back much of the welfare state through neoliberal restructuring and fiscal austerity, and thus it did not privilege rollout manoeuvres such as developing sector-wide P3 programs to promote partnerships with the private sector. This would change in 1999 with the creation of the SuperBuild infrastructure plan, and this initiative stands as the Harris government's attempt to institutionalize P3 development. However, with decision-making housed within the Cabinet Committee on Privatization and SuperBuild and few systematized capital planning procedures, this proto-enabling field remained far too politicized and lacked the routines necessary to sufficiently transform government operations and normalize P3 use. Nonetheless it did lead to the initiation of the province's first two P3 hospitals. From a P3-proponent perspective, SuperBuild can be considered a disappointment relative to the Liberals' Alternative Financing and Procurement (AFP) strategy – though this was far from obvious at the time.

The intention to use a P3 to deliver the Brampton Civic Hospital and Royal Ottawa Hospital projects was announced in November 2001, and

---

1 Mike Harris served as premier from 1995 to 1999 and was re-elected in 1999. Ernie Eves (PC) held this position from April 2002 to October 2003 after Harris stepped down.

by 2002 both requests for proposals had been issued. In 2001 Brampton was to be a roughly 700-bed facility and Ottawa was to have a little fewer than 300 beds. Correspondingly, the Ottawa project was to cost far less: an estimated $95 million in 2001 versus nearly $400 million estimated for Brampton in that same year.

These P3s received heavy criticism and much publicized concern, with resistance directed mainly by public sector unions and public health care advocates, though the Brampton hospital initially received more attention as a result of its much larger size. By September 2003 both projects were fiercely targeted by a coalition of union/public service advocacy groups (the Canadian Union of Public Employees, CUPE; the Ontario Public Service Employees Union, OPSEU; and the Ontario Health Coalition, OHC) which launched a court injunction to stop the proposed deals and the proposed Centre for Mental Health and Addiction in Toronto. The group claimed that P3 hospitals violated the Canada Health Act and provincial Public Hospitals Act, but ultimately their case was rejected by the Court for lack of sufficient evidence ("Unions Lose Bid" 2003). Other tactics were employed, including a four-year legal battle to gain access to financial details and other information surrounding the Brampton P3. Eventually details were released on the project agreement and lenders' agreement, but some crucial information has yet to be made public (Ontario Standing Committee on Government Agencies 2008). The NDP also sought details through freedom of information requests but received documents so heavily redacted that they were of little use – except, of course, that this is a clear example of the secrecy that accompanies P3s and the arduous nature of the fight against privatization.

Civil society–led resistance was also matched with politicization through partisan policy debate. During the spring and summer of 2003, McGuinty was steadfast in his efforts to distance himself and his party from the PCs' P3 agenda. Typical promises made during this part of the election campaign were that McGuinty would "dismantle" these agreements if he came to power (Blackwell 2003). Once it became clear that the Liberals would likely be forming government after the October election, in September 2003 McGuinty affirmed that these much-needed projects would still go forward, though not as "P3s," stating that P3s "represent an extraordinary departure from our history when it comes to public hospitals in the province of Ontario" and therefore the projects would be brought "back within the public system" (Lindgren 2003, 1).

When the McGuinty victory finally came, P3-related election promises were only partially fulfilled, given the nearly identical features of P3 and AFP hospital projects (see chapter 5). SuperBuild was replaced by the Liberals' new Ministry of Public Infrastructure Renewal (which would later house Infrastructure Ontario), and Alternative Financing and Procurement (AFP) rules and routines were introduced through the Infrastructure Planning, Financing, and Procurement Framework (IPFP). Thus the P3-enabling field as it stands today was put in place over the first few years that followed the election. This has allowed infrastructure P3s to proliferate in key sectors such as health and transportation to an extent that may not have been possible under the PC government, given the degree of resistance and politicization witnessed from 2001 to 2003. What became of the province's pioneering P3 hospitals is also a testament to the commitment that the Liberals have shown to private for-profit involvement in the public health care system: project agreement lengths were shortened, project scope was changed, and public ownership of the land and facilities was reasserted, but aside from these aspects, both went forward as full-spectrum design, build, finance, operate (DBFO) P3s.

The Liberals inherited an unexpected $5.6 billion deficit in November 2003, which some say forced them to not entirely scrap the P3 deals – not only because the government now "needed" the private financing but also because reneging on these deals would have cost the government an estimated $10 million (Hill 2003, 1; McArthur 2003). While these arguments do have some merit, the subsequent proliferation of P3 hospitals under the Liberals discredits any notion that they were not on board with P3s from the start. Furthermore, the $10 million penalty was later revealed to be only $2 million (OPSEU 2007, 6).

History

The roots of the Brampton Civic Hospital project run deep, with the first steps towards a new hospital being taken in 1971 when the Chinguacousy County Council voted to buy twenty hectares of land and dedicated the use of this lot to a future public hospital (Keung 2003). Since there was only one hospital in the immediate area at the time (Peel Memorial), when the population in Brampton began to swell – increasing by nearly 20 per cent between 1981 and 1985 alone – so too did the need for a new hospital.

By as early as 1984 the lack of public funding had the district health council entertaining notions of allowing a privately built hospital to be established on the site in order to fulfil this need

(McMonagle 1984).[2] During the 1985 provincial election campaign, Liberal party leader David Peterson promised that if he was elected premier he would make building a second hospital in the region a "major priority" for his Cabinet (Barker 1986). Peterson won the election but this promise was never honoured and the project languished in the proposal stage for years. In 1986 the Chinguacousy Health Services Centre Board, formed in 1973 to develop plans for a second hospital in the region, submitted their proposal to the province for a new 300-bed hospital in Brampton (Steen 1986), but by 1991 the project was not only stalled, it had been scaled down to a far more limited crisis centre and drop-in clinic to accommodate the lack of public spending (Mitchell 1991). Frustrated by decades-long inertia, in 1991 Brampton mayor Peter Robertson requested that if the newly elected Bob Rae NDP government was "unable to assist us at this time, then please set us free to negotiate with private interests for this health care centre" (Funston 1991). Despite the appeal and the clear need for a new hospital in the region, neither public nor private plans went forward.

Later that decade, in 1997, the Health Services Restructuring Commission[3] (HSRC) decided that the three hospital boards in the region (governing the Georgetown and District Memorial Hospital, Etobicoke General Hospital, and Peel Memorial Hospital) should be amalgamated under the newly created William Osler Health Centre (WOHC) (then known as the Northwest GTA Hospital Corporation), becoming the province's sixth-largest public health corporation. At the same time, the HSRC reaffirmed the need for a new hospital in the Brampton region and decided that the Peel Memorial Hospital should also be renovated and redeveloped. By late 2001, provincial finance minister Jim Flaherty and health minister Tony Clement had announced that the Brampton project would go forward as a P3 (Boyle 2001). The new hospital was to be built alongside the redevelopment of the Peel Memorial Hospital, the latter being slated to gain an additional 112 beds

---

2 District Health Councils (DHCs) were the predecessor of the Local Health Integration Networks (LHIN). Prior to 2005, DHCs provided advice to the Ministry of Health, informing them of local needs. DHCs were dissolved in advance of the creation of LHINs.

3 The HSRC was established by the Progressive Conservatives in 1996 to advise the Ministry of Health on decisions relating to "restructuring Ontario's public hospitals ... [and] on other aspects of Ontario's health services system" (Ontario Auditor General 2008, 108).

using traditional public financing and procurement (OHC 2008, 3). The P3 project eventually went through, but the redevelopment of Peel Memorial was later scrapped and by 2007 health services at Peel Memorial were discontinued and transferred (along with 234 patients) to the newly built Brampton Civic Hospital.

First opening its doors in 1910, the Royal Ottawa Hospital (then known as the Lady Grey Hospital) initially treated tuberculosis patients but by the early 1960s had begun to focus on mental health and psychiatric disorders (The Royal n.d.). By the late 1980s many problems were beginning to crop up with this facility as, for instance, overcrowding began to emerge (e.g., Dyer 1987), and leaks, cramped spaces, and a functionally obsolete design were growing concerns. In addition, in 1997 the HSRC announced that 140 patients would be transferred from a Brockville mental health facility to the Royal Ottawa Hospital by 1999, with $11 million suggested for renovations to accommodate this transfer; no additional funding was earmarked for improving the already cramped conditions and increasingly decrepit facility (Schliesmann 1997; Denley 2000). Separate redevelopment plans were thus initiated by the hospital board in 1999, although this was made public only in May 2000 when it announced that negotiations had begun with the provincial government to demolish the facility and replace it with a new $85 million hospital (ibid.). This "brownfield" proposal to build a new facility on an existing site was purported to be more economical than simply renovating the old facility, a less desirable option since the hospital board estimated that a new facility would cost $4 million less a year to run (ibid.).[4] Announced at the same time as the Brampton P3, in November 2001 the province committed to building a new 284 bed Royal Ottawa Hospital from the ground up, using a P3. One interviewee (public partner manager 5, interview, 15 October 2012) reported that without private funding, it would have taken roughly ten years to receive funding from the province, given the many projects already in line. Perhaps for reasons of expediency, the hospital's chief executive George Langill was an enthusiastic supporter of the P3 approach from the start (Egan 2001).

---

4 Brownfield projects are new facilities built on existing sites, whereas greenfield projects involve the construction of new facilities on newly selected sites. The Diamond Centre and Royal Ottawa P3s are examples of the former, while the Abbotsford and Brampton hospital P3s are examples of the latter.

Initiation

When both P3s were announced in late 2001, the justifications for deviating from the traditional method varied. Initially health minister Tony Clement promoted P3s as being "faster, better, and cheaper" (e.g., Lindgren 2001; "Ontario Health Minister" 2002). Critics were quick to point out that P3s rarely save the government money, given the presence of a profit motive and the higher interest rates paid by private borrowers, and finance minister Jim Flaherty shifted the debate away from absolute cost into the more opaque realm of efficiency and value for money (Boyle 2001).

The resolve to use P3s to deliver these hospitals clearly did not rest on an established track record, given the earlier problems with P3s in the province, nor was it based on the merits of each individual case, since the Ministry of Finance had announced six months earlier that P3s would have to be first considered before the government would commit to funding any new hospital projects (Ontario Auditor General 2008, 102). This bias was also made clear in a Ministry of Health and Long-Term Care (MOHLTC) letter sent to the WOHC in February 2002 that "directed that the P3 model must be the one used for the development of the new [Brampton] hospital, and that other options or deviations from this model could not be considered" (108). The government was promising that these pioneering projects would be "the first of many," and it was hoping to extend the model into all feasible sectors, "from hospitals to hockey rinks" (Boyle 2001).

Once the government announced in November 2001 that it would be launching these P3s, the various bidding stages were quickly initiated in early 2002, which allowed for little public input and deliberation. Private input, on the other hand, was solicited.

With the Brampton project the prospective private partners were given significant latitude to mould the P3 as they wished. For instance, rather than the public sector dictating the parameters of the project agreement, at the Request for Expression of Interest stage in March 2002 bidders were asked "to state their interest in contracting for *some* or *all* of the necessary work ("William Osler Health Centre" 2002, emphasis added). The government then required that the WOHC compare the price of private sector bids to the cost of delivering a fully public hospital (Ontario Auditor General 2008, 104). As the WOHC assessment was merely a reference point and not a full business case, P3 value for money was never truly established, and the private proponents' bids largely guided the comparison and decision-making.

Private consultants were also relied upon, especially once the bidding and negotiation stages began. As reported by the provincial auditor general, the WOHC and MOHLTC hired nearly sixty legal, technical, and financial consultants at a cost of $34 million (with $6 million incurred prior to the government's decision to use a P3, and $28 million once this route was chosen) (Ontario Auditor General 2008, 105). Not only were these costs not added to the price of the P3, but the use of multiple private consultancy firms produced a wide variety of estimates – leading to confusion, criticism, and misinformed public debate later on. One of the first consulting firms hired by the WOHC (September 2000, prior to the decision to use a P3) estimated that the traditional procurement method would cost roughly $357 million. In October 2001 this was updated to $381 million. Another private consulting firm (commissioned in January 2003) came up with a much larger figure: $507 million, which was updated to $525 million in November 2004. Not only did the hospital board "not question the large difference in the two estimates," but Ontario's auditor general also noted that these figures greatly overestimated the cost of the traditional method (2010, 306). Cost creep and changes in estimated costs such as those seen with all four P3 hospitals examined here are borne by the public. Capital costs are locked in and subject to risk transfer provisions only once P3 project agreements are signed.

The actions and decision-making procedures of the public sector demonstrate the lack of routinization and in-house expertise at the time. In contrast to AFP routines where the functional plan and project's scope and size are set out ahead of the decision to use a P3 and three standardized value for money stages occur during procurement, the steps taken with the Brampton hospital suggest little forethought went into the public sector role. These steps are summarized by the auditor general (2008, 114–15): in January 2003 the WOHC came up with its initial estimate of what the hospital would cost if a traditional public approach was used, which was almost a year after the request for proposals had been issued. This value for money estimate should have instead been the basis upon which the P3 route was pursued in the first place. The WOHC updated this estimate two years later, in November 2004, after the preferred bidder had already been chosen. Meanwhile, the MOHLTC was conducting its own reviews of the WOHC's analyses, the first being finalized after the request for proposals stage was complete, and the second (which, remarkably, the WOHC was unaware of) was finished in 2005 after the project agreement had been struck. Though each phase confirmed the superiority of the P3 route, using a

P3 appears to have been a fait accompli from the start, no matter what the results. Furthermore, the auditor general has since discredited all of these value for money calculations (to be addressed in the next section), leading one to reasonably question whether intentional manipulation rather than mere error had occurred.

With the Royal Ottawa Hospital, the choice to use a P3 was also made prior to establishing value for money, but this decision was reached in a way very different way from that of the Brampton hospital. First the hospital board (the Royal Ottawa Health Care Group, ROHCG) sought and was awarded approval through SuperBuild to begin the P3; next, the ROH Project Implementation Management Team issued a formal request for proposals, selected from among the bidders, and later came to form the public partner. Thus, unlike with the WOHC, it was the public hospital board (ROHCG) that largely drove the process of using a P3. This is consistent with the ROHCG's previous track record of enthusiasm for support service privatization – it was among the first in Ontario to contract out non-clinical care (1995), slashing staff numbers nearly in half in order to save money. Laird and Langill (2005, 71), lead consultant to the ROHCG and former CEO of the ROHCG respectively, explain that – given the combination of prior experience with contracting-out, a supportive hospital board, and the recent creation of SuperBuild – "the timing was right to consider this [P3] approach in the healthcare arena." The board's justifications for the P3 followed the familiar refrain of saving money, building the facility more quickly, and improving staff and patient well-being (ROMHC 2003). Each justification has since been shown to bear no correspondence with the reality of this project (to be addressed in the next section).

Bidding and negotiation occurred during 2002 and 2003, and were kept highly secretive. The opaque nature of this process was excused by the ROHCG at the time on the grounds that confidentiality would "ensure fairness and a strong competitive process" (ROMHC 2003, 30). Indicative of the lack of routinization under SuperBuild, the steps taken to deliver this project differ significantly from the Brampton experience. Laird and Langill (2005) describe the major steps that they took, and how they came to these decisions. After deciding to use a P3, the ROHCG prepared a very limited functional program in hopes that giving the private partner significant leeway would lead to superior designs. The board also recognized that a P3 would require "a major realignment of our governance and management resources" so experts (including an experienced project manager) were sought out to provide financial, technical, and legal assistance, and the board created the Expansion and Redevelopment Committee to oversee the entire process (72). Even if this helped improve the development of the P3, these experts were never called on to judge whether a P3 should be used; and between the hospital board's commitment to privatization and the embedded involvement of leading P3 market actors, conflict of interest and bias were almost certainly present.

The committee then produced a value for money benchmark, which was used to evaluate bids; however, it was also disclosed to the bidders at the request-for-proposals stage. Allowing those bidding to see this information effectively squashed the competitive pressure needed to ensure that proposals were as cost-effective as possible. Two bidding stages then followed (request for qualifications and request for proposals), running throughout most of 2002 and 2003. Shortly after the negotiations with the preferred bidder had begun, the provincial election took place in October 2003.

Having yet to reach commercial and financial close, the newly elected McGuinty government forced through several changes prior to signing the Royal Ottawa Hospital project agreement in July 2004. They included shortening the length of the agreement from what would have likely been sixty-six years to twenty-one years (Adam 2003), and amending the legal arrangements pertaining to ownership of the facility and land (putting these elements back in public hands). The analogy used by the CEO of the ROHCG, George Langille, to characterize the change in ownership provisions was that it amounted to the difference between leasing a house and taking out a mortgage to finance the purchasing of a house (Adam 2004). As Langille describes the changes that McGuinty's government imposed, "There is no question that you have a public ownership component that you didn't have before" (ibid.). These are certainly improvements on the more egregious aspects of initial P3 arrangements, but the NDP were also right when they pointed out at the time that "whether it is a lease or mortgage, the private consortium will still make the usual 20-per-cent profit – money that will be 'siphoned off patient care to big private companies'" (quoted in ibid.).

Value for Money?

In 2001, Ontario's finance minister pegged the cost of building the Brampton hospital at roughly $350 million, to begin in 2002 ("Ontario Plans" 2001). Construction instead began in 2005 at a cost of $550 million – an increase of $200 million. And rather than opening in 2005, it began accepting patients in late 2007. This delay was due not only to the protracted nature of P3 negotiations; additional factors included the change in government and the lawsuit launched by CUPE, OPSEU, and the OHC. On the other hand, the auditor general noted that complications with finalizing the financial arrangements contributed to the delay, which certainly could be attributed to the P3 itself (Ontario Auditor General 2008, 115).

Cost increases have not corresponded to more beds; instead, capacity dropped from the September 2000 estimate of 716 to 479 beds in service when it first opened in 2007 (Ontario Auditor General 2008, 102–3). A full capacity of 608 beds was supposed to be reached in 2012, but by November 2012 the hospital had only 554 beds. It is possible that the failure to reach full capacity is not related to the P3 agreement but rather is the result of changes in the hospital's post-construction operating plan (decided by WOHC) (public partner manager 4, interview, 12 November 2012). Regardless, with the closure of the Peel Memorial Hospital came the elimination of the 112 beds promised with that redevelopment project, representing a significant net loss for the community. In 2003 the Regional Hospital Infrastructure Plan estimated that by 2008, 930 hospital beds would be required to adequately care for patients in the region (OHC 2008, 5).

The Royal Ottawa P3 suffers from similar shortcomings. Construction costs came in not at $95 million as promised by the health minister in 2001, but ended up amounting to $146 million (OPSEU 2007, 1). It also has fewer beds than the facility it replaced. Original estimates were for 284 beds, but it opened with nearly 100 fewer, for a total of 188. Delays plagued this P3. The PC government first suggested that the P3 route would speed up the process and estimated that completion would be achieved in May 2004 (Egan 2001), but the facility was operational only in 2006. Despite these problems, the P3 is touted as being "on time," "on budget" (e.g., Laird and Langill 2005, 79).

Value for money was not established ahead of time with either P3, thus the decision to use the P3 model could not have been based on P3 cost or value superiority. In Brampton the decision was also heavily skewed: the province overestimated the costs of traditional procurement by $289 million, which made the P3 option seem cheaper (Ontario Auditor General 2008, 114–17). This included overestimating design and construction costs and adding the costs associated with some non-clinical services that should not have been attributed to the public sector comparator (PSC) (104–5). The WOHC also incorrectly added

$67 million to its estimate of what a traditional hospital would cost as a way of accounting for the risk transfer that could be achieved with a P3. Yet the auditor general found that "a properly structured contract under a traditional procurement agreement could have mitigated any such cost overruns" (104). Thus a full spectrum DBFO P3 was not necessary, making these errors both mathematical and indicative of bias in favour of the P3. Furthermore, the higher price of private financing added an estimated $200 million over the lifetime of the project agreement (105). The interest rate spread was not considered when the WOHC compared the P3 to the traditional approach.

Scope and other related project changes that occurred after the project agreement was finalized led to additional costs incurred by the public partner, rather than being transferred to the private partner. This included a $63 million modification of the facility to accommodate equipment installation, owing to the disintegrated nature of P3 planning, which separates construction plans from equipment installation (Ontario Auditor General 2008, 116). Finally, hidden transaction costs not accounted for in the final price of the P3 (and thus borne entirely by the taxpayer) added an additional $28 million as a result of the large number of private advisors, consultants, and legal experts used (105). Despite all of these problems, the Brampton P3 has been labelled as being "on time," "on budget," and of "value" for taxpayers (e.g., "Construction Completed" 2007, 1).

Confirming or refuting value for money with respect to the Royal Ottawa Hospital is more difficult as there has been no public audit conducted – although data produced by economist Hugh Mackenzie are revealing. In 2005 he calculated that "if the hospital had been funded through government debt, the cost [of financing the capital and facility management services] in present value terms would have been $174 million lower" (quoted in Loxley 2010, 107). This is mainly the result of the higher interest rate paid by the private partner (6.33 per cent) (Adam 2009). Transaction costs have not been made public, but it is likely that they amounted to 10–12 per cent of the total costs.

These findings, along with construction costs coming in at over $50 million above what the P3 was originally supposed to cost, justify an audit. The call for involvement of the provincial auditor general gained even greater salience once the damning report on the Brampton hospital was released in late 2008. Public health care advocates and P3 critics have since been strongly advocating for this type of investigation. George Weber, president and CEO of the ROHCG, was more apathetic, arguing, "Infrastructure Ontario say they've learned some lessons from Brampton, so what's the use? Time has moved on" ("Audit on Royal Ottawa Sought" 2009). A public partner manager interviewed for this study echoed these sentiments – suggesting that with the creation of Infrastructure Ontario the process has been streamlined and changed significantly, thus if a P3 hospital were to be audited, it should be one developed under Infrastructure Ontario (public partner manager 5, interview, 15 October 2112). There can be no doubt that additional audits of P3 hospitals are needed in the province, yet these arguments hardly inspire confidence in the robustness of the value for money delivered by the Royal Ottawa P3. This stance also indicates that accountability and transparency remain poor.

Beyond the financial and methodological value for money details, value in terms of the quality of the building and equipment can be judged to be poor. Staff working within the Royal Ottawa Hospital have reported many significant problems with the building's design and the negative impact that it has had on patients, staff, and visitors (which is especially concerning given that it is a psychiatric facility), and the many problems that emerged within the first six months of its operation also challenge the notion that the project was in fact delivered "on time."

Problems ran the full gamut. There was an insufficient number of drinking water stations initially installed in the building, inadequate safety design in the reception area, poor air quality due to improper ventilation, ineffective sound insulation between clinical offices, unsuitable shower facilities, and difficult-to-operate doors to wards in the geriatric unit (OPSEU 2007; Adam 2008). Equipment failures were also significant, particularly those related to security. They included problems with the security cameras, malfunctioning wireless technology (including telephones, fax machines, and switchboard operations), a lack of handheld panic buttons and sterilization equipment, security breaches and patient escapes due to a lack of security (ibid.). George Weber called these "teething problems" and suggested they had nothing to do with the use of a P3 (Adam 2009). This was also one of the first hospitals in Canada with a wireless environment (including fax machines, security cameras, etc.), and most issues were resolved satisfactorily by the private partner within six months. However, even if one agrees that these types of problems could occur with any new hospital, particularly one using new technology, the speed and effectiveness with which labour-related issues in particular have been addressed was less than stellar. For staff working in a P3 hospital, the internal bifurcation of authority, to be examined in the section that follows, presents its own unique challenges.

Private Partners, Private Services

In his 2008 report on the Brampton Civic Hospital P3, the provincial auditor general expressed concern that the government had not conducted a market assessment in order to gauge whether there was sufficient construction-sector capacity and the competitive pressure needed to generate the best bids possible. Had a market assessment been conducted, it would have become apparent that, in the auditor's words, "only a limited number of construction contractors in the province [were] able or willing to undertake a project of this size. The same construction companies would be involved in the bidding and work regardless of whether WOHC followed the traditional procurement or P3 approach" (2008, 108). These findings are equally applicable to the Royal Ottawa Hospital project. Both requests for proposals generated three bids, but a lack of competition and capacity overall led to a situation where the identical consortium formed the private partner for both project agreements.

The Brampton Civic Hospital's 2005 winning bid came from a consortium named The Healthcare Infrastructure Company of Canada (THICC). THICC designed, built, and financed the infrastructure, and since 2007 holds a twenty-five-year non-clinical support service contract (including laundry, housekeeping, patient portering, security, maintenance, and dietary services). THICC is a partnership between Canadian construction giant EllisDon, Borealis Capital Ltd (the investment arm of the Ontario Municipal Employees Retirement System, a public sector pension fund), and Carillion Canada Inc (a subsidiary of the United Kingdom's Carillion, a longstanding P3 market actor providing infrastructure support services). Architectural design was provided by Parkin Architects and Adamson Associates Architects of Toronto. Similarly, in 2004 THICC was awarded the contract to design, build, finance, maintain, and operate the Royal Ottawa Hospital. Upon its opening in 2006, there has been a twenty-one-year non-clinical service agreement in place.

Small and medium-sized contractors in Ontario have expressed concern with the monopolization of P3 markets by large firms. This problem is generated at least in part through AFP rules that stipulate that financial risks are transferred to all members of the winning consortium – meaning that even the construction firm has to qualify for surety insurance, bonding, and parent company guarantees that may not be available to smaller contractors (Ontario Standing Committee on Government Agencies 2008). Another problem, and one that is shared by small contractors in all P3 markets, is the essence of the P3 approach: contract bundling. Proponents claim that bundling allows for innovation and efficiencies to be generated by P3s, but it is also the main feature that reduces competition overall, since it increases risk, the timeline for development, and the costs taken on by the companies that form the private partner. Mike Sharp, chairman of the Ottawa Construction Association, argued that for trade contractors the risk profile with DBFOs is extremely high, estimating this to be two times greater than what would be present with large, traditional projects (Ontario Standing Committee on Government Agencies 2008). He also estimated that AFP bidding procedures are nearly four times as expensive as they are with traditional bidding (ibid.). Thus while P3 profitability for private partners is produced mainly by taking on risks that do not materialize, only relatively secure and well-capitalized firms can operate successfully in this niche. By 2012 it was still only the largest construction companies – PCL and EllisDon in particular – that were active participants in Ontario's P3 hospital market (see Infrastructure Ontario n.d.).

Private governance-related concerns arising from these pioneering P3 hospitals relate to three important issues: the length, breadth, and bundling of contracts; the internal bifurcation of authority (including commercialization); and the reduced accountability that accompanies their use. Even though several important aspects of the Brampton and Ottawa project agreements were changed for the better after the 2003 election (e.g., alterations made to ownership provisions and reduced contract lengths), all P3 hospitals suffer from problems related to their partially privatized mode of hospital governance.

The Ontario Health Coalition prepared a list summarizing how the features of the Brampton P3 went well beyond earlier forms of privatization in Ontario's public health care system: support service privatization was far longer than ever before (more than twenty years), and contracts involved a wider range of services; bundling support services with all other project elements was completely novel; the project agreement allowed the private for-profit partner unprecedented rights to develop commercial ventures inside and around the hospital; and no previous agreement had ever allowed the private partner to sell its interest in the project after the agreement was signed (OHC 2008, 9).[5] This list applies to the Royal Ottawa Hospital as well, with one caveat being that support-service privatization had already taken place in that hospital in 1995.[6]

Within both hospitals, the private partner (THICC) controls and oversees the management and operation of all non-clinical services. This is referred to as an "internal bifurcation of authority," given that the hospital board is no longer responsible for, nor does it control, this part of the hospital's operations. Shrybman (2007) argues that there are two important problems that arise from this arrangement: first, it can negatively affect health-service delivery and efficiencies, since the integration of non-clinical and clinical patient care is vital to hospital operations; and second, the bundling of all non-clinical service contracts puts financial pressure on the hospital board, given that these payments come from uncertain future budgets. With the Brampton hospital, for example, the facility's lease payments are covered by the province, but the service contract is not. In lean years the hospital board may be pressured into allowing greater hospital commercialization, given that these costs amount to roughly half of the WOHC's hospital budget over the length of project agreement (OHC 2008, 9).

The effects of this internal bifurcation of authority were made especially visible within the first few years of the Royal Ottawa's operations. As mentioned earlier, the many significant concerns that emerged with the building's design and equipment functionality not only negatively affected patients, staff, and visitors but also raised the issue of who is actually accountable and responsible for decision-making in this P3 hospital. The union representing staff within the hospital reported that the "lines of accountability and authority have become blurred" (OPSEU 2007, 2) and that clarifying which partner is actually accountable for particular tasks is difficult to achieve, since managers are not allowed to view any of the contracts and "are simply expected to accept the word of Carillion managers with respect to entitlements" (14). This can

---

5 While equity sales are permissible, refinancing (another major concern associated with P3-related financialization) may occur only with the prior approval of the WOHC, and the WOHC must receive half of all refinancing gains (Loxley 2010, 110).

6 Johnson Controls held these contracts, and the employees were simply transferred over to Carillion when the P3 began. In the 1990s provincial wage-settlement agreements ensured that CUPE-organized staff working for Johnson Controls were paid roughly the same as CUPE-organized public sector workers (public partner manager 5, interview, 15 October 2012).

lead to a tense work environment for staff because, as one union member described it, "everything is a fight" (14). Lack of transparency and accountability also raise the concern that health services might be threatened. For example, the union claims that maintenance costs have been downloaded onto clinical program budgets since "hospital program budgets are billed for damage/maintenance considered by Carillion not to be due to 'normal use'" (2).

Concerns continue to emerge. In 2011 an issue arose surrounding which partner picks up the cost associated with the administrative dietician who oversees food services provided by Carillion. This position is supposed to be covered by Carillion, but it is possible that Carillion changed the job title to avoid this cost (R. Janson, campaigns officer, OPSEU interview, 22 June 2012).

Labour relations in Ontario's public health care system differ from the situation in BC in two important respects: contracting-out has been far less extensive (there is currently no legislation akin to BC's Bill 29-2002) and, related to the former, health care support staff receive similar wages in Ontario's public and private sectors. The 1997 Public Sector Labour Relations Transition Act (PSLRTA) essentially allows workers to take their contract with them – if work is contracted-out, the terms and conditions set in the public sector are applied to the private contractor. Thus terms and conditions are roughly identical for hospital staff working in P3 settings and traditional settings (D. Allan, researcher, OCHU, interview, 18 July 2012). Without a significant reduction in labour costs associated with contracting-out, privatization efforts are stymied.

Observations

Ontario's change in government in 2003 held important consequences for its first P3 hospitals and future P3s developed in the province. They include subsequent implementation of its enabling field in 2004 and 2005, composed primarily of a capital planning framework (AFP and the Infrastructure Planning Financing and Procurement Framework, IPFP) and a specialized government agency dedicated to P3 development (Infrastructure Ontario). Given the timing of these developments, both the Brampton Civic Hospital and the Royal Ottawa Hospital were largely unaffected by the routines, institutional support, and depoliticization offered by the Liberal enabling field. In both cases negotiations with the preferred bidder were nearly complete just prior to the 2003 election, but the project agreements had not yet been finalized. On the basis of available evidence, one may reasonably conclude that the changes implemented by the Liberals were of some benefit to health care users, hospital workers, and taxpayers. For instance, had these P3s project agreements not been renegotiated by the Liberals, they would have been decades longer and contained additional elements of privatization (i.e., private ownership of land and facilities). Features such as these exacerbated value for money and governance concerns.

However, it is also important to not overstate the degree to which these P3s (and those that followed) were altered by AFP and the rest of the enabling field. The main difference between the model of public-private partnerships established by the PC government and the Liberal version is that with the latter the facilities and land remain in public hands – and this is basis upon which Liberals claim that their AFP model is not a "P3" (e.g., Ontario Ministry of Infrastructure 2011). But this claim ignores many other essential similarities: project agreements remain decades-long and the design, building, financing, and operating of the infrastructure is conducted by for-profit private partners. Further, whether these hospitals will one day be fully public remains to be seen. No evidence suggests that once P3 project agreements expire several decades from now, operation and maintenance services will be returned to the public sector. In fact the full-scale privatization of the Highway 407 P3 suggests that P3s can also open the door to more permanent forms of privatization.

Having been initiated during the SuperBuild era, the controversy and problems experienced with the pioneering P3s examined here can be attributed, at least in part, to the failures of this proto-enabling field. The experience taught proponents two main lessons. First, it guided the subsequent development of a sector-wide P3 program in health care. This P3 program now focuses exclusively on large infrastructure development (i.e., projects above $20 million), conducted with the support of Infrastructure Ontario – smaller projects have entirely different funding streams and procurement protocols. Infrastructure-procurement innovations occurred for both traditional and P3 projects, securing the P3 niche in the health sector. Second, it helped mould the Liberal AFP approach, its emphasis on public ownership of land and facilities, and the development of P3 routines (more on the AFP "difference" in the subsequent section). Thus the failures of Ontario's initial P3 hospitals were used not, as one might suppose, to justify a return to traditional procurement but instead firmed up a role for P3s in the area of large hospital infrastructure development and helped to improve routinization, institutionalization, and depoliticization of the P3 model overall.

One major contradiction of the SuperBuild era, revealed in different ways through both hospital cases, relates to the problems that can arise when ideologically driven Cabinet-level decision-making unfolds without the support of routines and institutions that can help smooth out and depoliticize the process. The decision to use a P3 in both cases was made by government simply on the basis that the private sector *ought* to be involved – that it would be inherently less costly, quicker, and better to do so. Yet the responsibility for carrying out most stages of development was shifted onto the shoulders of inexperienced hospital boards.

With the Brampton Civic Hospital the lack of P3 procurement routines and value for money expertise led to several errors and missteps along the way. First, it meant that the costs of traditional procurement were vastly overestimated (by $289 million), allowing the P3 option to be presented as being cheaper when in fact it was of worse value for money. This methodological error indicates not only bias but also the difficulty that an inexperienced agency can have when carrying out this important role. The use of different private consultants' reports to establish value for money at various stages of procurement was also a disorganized process and led to many different cost estimates and multiple revisions. Under AFP these processes have been standardized and made uniform across projects and sectors, though this has not necessarily led to better value for money, as the next section on proliferation will discuss.

With the Royal Ottawa Hospital, procurement stages appear to have been well structured by the hospital board, but the process suffered from a high level of secrecy, which led to greater civil-society resistance. Transparency has been improved with the creation of Infrastructure Ontario, as it posts bidding information and documents related to projects and value for money on its website. Yet here too concerns persist. More information and greater predictability has not translated into substantially improved transparency, given the significant redactions and lack of financial data contained in the documents provided to the public.

The low level of expertise, routines, and standardization also led to problems with the operational phase of these projects. With the Brampton case this takes the form of a service agreement that is difficult to monitor and with the Royal Ottawa Hospital it has led to accountability issues. One of the most significant changes made to Ontario's health sector P3 program was therefore the December 2006 Ministry of Health and Long-Term Care exclusion of soft facility services such as laundry, linen, patient portering, housekeeping, and food services from future P3 hospital deals. This does not mean that soft services cannot be privatized through contracting-out, but they can no longer be bundled within a P3 project agreement. Hard facility services that encompass day-to-day management of a hospital such as heating, electricity, lighting, security, and parking are still included in P3 deals.

Performance of support-service providers at the Brampton Civic Hospital reflects this division. One interviewee reports that hard facility services have "been performing fine," whereas with soft facility services "it has been variable" – in particular, there are problems exist with discharge cleaning and portering (public partner manager 4, interview, 12 November 2012). However, a penalty has not yet been applied. Non-patient food, parking, and security have been subcontracted by Carillion, and the security vendor has been changed as the result of poor performance. A private partner manager interviewed for this study supports the decision to exclude most soft services: "There needs to be a reason to put [services in] ... why would you have patient food services in the model? It's 35 per cent food costs and 45 per cent labour. It doesn't matter how long the contract is ... I don't see what you get by adding that in" (private partner manager 1, interview, 29 October 2012). In contrast, this private partner manager suggests that transferring risk for hard facility services (and the interviewee includes housekeeping in this category) to the private partner ensures that once a project agreement has expired, the facility is returned to the public partner in good working order.

The wider implications of this exemption for the P3 model are more complex. On the one hand it is a positive development since it reduces concerns about the internal bifurcation of authority – but it does not entirely eliminate these problems given that many hard facility services (such as the helpdesk, upkeep of electrical and HVAC systems) are also important to hospital service planning and management. On the other hand, even though this was a victory for P3 opponents, it has also extended the longevity of the model. As Ron Sapsford, deputy health minister, put it, the decision was made to exclude these services "because of the operating difficulties that can arise ... [and] leaving those services out simplifies substantially the contractual understandings and agreements that have to be put into place" (Ontario Standing Committee on Public Accounts 2009). To the extent that the major concerns of those most vocally opposed to P3 hospitals have been neutralized, P3s are able to flourish now more than ever in the public health care sector.

The SuperBuild era also suffered from thinly institutionalized P3 policy. The Cabinet Committee on Privatization and SuperBuild could have potentially developed into a centre of expertise and method of institutionalization like Infrastructure Ontario, but this had not taken place prior to the 2003 election. Neither pioneering hospital therefore benefited from the support provided by a specialized government agency dedicated to promoting and developing P3s. With the creation of Infrastructure Ontario, the provincial health sector P3 program was solidified. However, institutionalization has occurred without any systematic evaluation of whether the track record of these initial projects warranted their future use, and the Liberals sought very little public input. Natalie Mehra, director of the Ontario Health Coalition, reported that the invitation-only consultations that informed the creation of Infrastructure Ontario were held mainly with P3 market participants, and "all the questions were about how to do P3s, not whether or not to do P3s" (Ontario Standing Committee on Government Agencies 2008).

P3s were also institutionalized as the de facto standard model of large hospital development without any prior evaluation of traditional project success. When asked whether he had ever been required to conduct an analysis of the history of traditional procurement in the province (i.e., how many hospitals were delivered on time, on budget, etc.), David Livingston, president and CEO of Infrastructure Ontario in 2008, confirmed that this type of assessment had never been done (Ontario Standing Committee on Government Agencies 2008). The track record of the traditional model was therefore not the basis on which the decision to use P3s in Ontario's health sector was made, again revealing the ideological nature of this policy.

Proliferation

Ontario's health sector has become the major target of P3 development in the province. This has been accomplished through the creation of an enabling field and its routinization, institutionalization, and depoliticization of private for-profit involvement within the system. These efforts may have made P3s more palatable but have they actually improved the P3 model and project success? Some glaring problems have certainly been smoothed out through standardization and public sector expertise building, but several core concerns remain. In particular, the AFP program has led to the flourishing of P3s without substantial improvement in transparency and value for money.

Reflecting on the auditor general's criticisms of the Brampton Civic Hospital project, public officials representing the hospital board, Infrastructure Ontario, and Ministry of Health assured the public at a Standing Committee on Public Accounts hearing held in 2009 that early P3s are significantly different from AFP today. In addition to the principle of public ownership, the standardization of value for money procedures is held up as a central benefit of the AFP model today (Ontario Standing Committee on Public Accounts 2009). Each new project is now subjected to three value for money assessments at different stages of development, and Infrastructure Ontario provides technical assistance along the way. The presence of a P3 unit and procurement routines avoids the use of multiple private consultants (eliminating contradictory cost estimates) and reliance upon ill-equipped hospital boards to assess value for money. The results of these assessments are also made available online through Infrastructure Ontario's website, supposedly increasing transparency.

On the surface it would appear that the process has improved greatly. Delving deeper, several problems emerge. First, value for money is derived mainly through risk transfer. This is made clear in Infrastructure Ontario's *Value for Money* manual, which demonstrates that base costs, financing costs, and transaction costs are actually lower for the public sector comparator. Yet justifying a P3 on the basis of risk transfer alone is highly problematic, since it assumes that a well-designed traditional contract will not be able to adequately mitigate risk. Second, specific to AFP, Infrastructure Ontario's risk-transfer matrices appear to have been institutionalized without rigorous confirmation of their methodology (Loxley 2012). Third, when private consultants are hired by Infrastructure Ontario to "independently" verify value for money, they do not actually "audit or attempt to verify the accuracy or completeness of the information or assumptions underlying the [public sector comparator]," leading Loxley (2012, 22) to ask, "What exactly are they doing?" Fourth, risk estimates are extremely sensitive – even modest changes made to the estimates of public and private sector costs produce significant differences. Sheila Block (2008) recalculated the value for money offered by fourteen of Ontario's more recent P3 (AFP) hospitals using "more realistic assumptions about public/private cost differentials" and, "rather than saving the province $341 million as Infrastructure Ontario calculations show, these projects cost the province an additional $585 million for a net difference of $926 million" (5).

Results such as these are alarming but difficult to substantiate because of the second major unresolved problem with AFP: the level of disclosure and transparency remains so low that it is impossible for the public to definitively recalculate value for money. Documents available online are missing critical financial information.

AFP was supposed to have fixed the problems of the earlier P3 process, but for many of the most significant concerns improvements have been more rhetorical than real. AFP has been characterized as a better way of delivering value for money, transferring risk, and ensuring transparency, given the Infrastructure Planning, Financing, and Procurement Framework (IPFP) recognition of principles such as ensuring the public interest and a transparent process, and demonstrating value for money. However, there is no legislation to actually guarantee that IPFP principles are upheld with each P3. In fact the case study evidence indicates that the public interest, value for money, transparency, and accountability are all *undermined* by P3s. Shifting P3 selection into the realm of the technocracy thus misleads the electorate while offering no real protection for the public interest. An editorial in the *Toronto Star* ("Dubious Financing for Health Facility" 2005) nicely summarizes the situation by stating that the Liberals' AFP is "just another name for the unloved P3s, public-private partnerships, first introduced by the former Conservative government of Mike Harris and Ernie Eves."

Concluding Remarks

Much like in BC, Ontario's initial P3 hospitals were highly politicized, offered poor value for money, and came in much later and at a higher price than originally promised. Aside from these similarities, there is one major difference: their timing on the creation of the wider provincial enabling field. In BC, P3 hospitals were developed together with the enabling field, while in Ontario the first P3 hospitals were initiated several years prior. A related difference is the political upheaval caused by the Ontario provincial election (October 2003), which occurred well after these projects were first announced (November 2001). This greatly increased the level of policy debate, public awareness, and need for strong and overt support by Cabinet (and the premier in particular) to push these deals through to completion. For all these reasons, critics had a relatively louder voice in Ontario than in BC.

The Brampton Civic Hospital and Royal Ottawa Hospital were the first in a long and ever-growing line of P3 hospitals developed in Ontario. Without any prior examples within the province, it is understandable that some mistakes and problems would have emerged with these pioneers. However, the number and magnitude of the issues that have since been uncovered are significant. Neither hospital was delivered on time or on budget, nor did these facilities provide a fully desirable level of functionality, design, and security/ well-being for patients and staff. Further, not only was value for money never established ahead of time, but serious methodological errors occurred along the way that erroneously supported the P3 option. Problems did not cease once they were operational, and these projects have remained the subject of much controversy. Worse still, these issues have not led to an abandonment of the policy but instead were used to guide the development of a sector-wide P3 program in health care.

The P3 health sector program initiated by the Liberals in the mid-2000s was designed to correct some obvious problems, but it also hid and/or ignored others. The role played by the pioneering projects was not to act as a yardstick for evaluating whether future P3s should be developed but instead to guide the unfolding of the enabling field. As the Brampton and Royal Ottawa cases demonstrate, if pragmatism were to trump ideology, then the opposition and internally generated problems with these first P3 hospitals should have put an end to experimentation with the model. Instead these projects helped to indicate where sources of resistance lay, and what types of market-like rules would be needed in the public sector in order to more successfully allow for privatization. Thus routinization and institutionalization have produced some improvements to P3 processes without substantially improving outcomes. Depoliticization has further normalized their use by obscuring the overtly ideological, political, and privatized nature of P3 projects. All things considered, despite a few relatively minor improvements made to the process of P3 development, the Ontario P3 enabling field has proven largely to enhance the appearance of P3 superiority whilst doing very little to address the essential pitfalls that accompany P3 projects.

Conclusion

The litany of problems associated with P3 projects suggests the potential for two types of crises with this model: crises of faith among policymakers (which is significant, given that ideological support for privatization remains crucial) and crises induced by internal contradictions. There is an obvious interrelation between the two as well, magnifying the potential for policy abandonment. For instance, P3s are touted as cost-saving instruments, but the empirical record demonstrates higher long-run expenses than traditional public procurement. Once P3s become the standard way in which large public infrastructure is provided, these additional cost burdens expand, and this may eventually make it more difficult to justify their use. Evidence of indefensibly higher P3 costs is emerging in the United Kingdom, the homeland of the model, and especially so within the health sector (e.g., Hope 2012; Alleyne 2012). As another example, the heart of P3 justification relates to risk transfer, yet many (new) risks are simultaneously created through reliance upon volatile financial markets and for-profit operators. P3 projects and policies are therefore in need of stabilization lest internal contradictions lead to collapsed deals and/or a rejection of the model by policymakers. Despite their higher economic and social costs, and the financial market turbulence in 2008–9, neither form of crisis has yet to truly emerge in Canada. P3s similarly continue to proliferate around the world. The theme of P3 policy stabilization, and how it occurs in light of these intrinsic problems, runs throughout this concluding chapter.

P3 Hospitals and Project Stabilization

Despite their growing popularity, P3 hospitals have proven unable to genuinely meet the expectations and promises of proponents. With all four cases examined here (the Abbotsford Regional Hospital and Cancer Centre, the Diamond Centre, the Brampton Civic Hospital, and the Royal Ottawa Hospital), bidding and negotiation delayed construction significantly, and cost creep occurred across the board. All four have nonetheless been labelled "on time and on budget," the purported reason being that once the project agreements were signed, these hospitals opened on schedule and without added cost to the public partner. However, this too is a stretch. There are two additional problems with these "on time and on budget" claims. First, P3 hospitals are not always completely functional when they first open. The Royal Ottawa Hospital had serious problems with its infrastructure and security, which took at least six months to remedy (including its wireless systems, and patient and staff facilities), and, by 2013, the Brampton Hospital was still not running at full capacity.

Second, how well risk was transferred, a central component of "on budget" and P3 value for money superiority claims, remains debatable. Changes made to the Diamond Centre's functionality after the project agreement was signed meant that key aspects of cost increase were borne solely by the public partner, and there are no provisions for withholding service payments in the case of poor private-partner performance. Similarly, changes made in the Brampton case also caused the public partner to bear the entire cost of items that were supposed to be transferred, and the service agreement is so complex that it is unclear whether the public partner is getting as much value out of the agreement as possible. The Abbotsford hospital agreement is more robust and ten of twelve services were to be provided by a new subcontractor in 2013 if they failed to meet performance expectations. However, this too indicates just how little risk is borne by the private partner, given that deductions and penalties are passed on to their subcontractors. Further, the Abbotsford public partner has proven unwilling to enforce payment-deduction provisions, rendering contractually based guarantees irrelevant. The rhetoric of P3s as mechanisms to insulate the public from project risks thus gives way to the reality that P3s reorient public sector decision-making by thoroughly incorporating the needs and interests of private partners.

The cases examined in chapters 5 and 6 also provide clear examples of methodological concerns (e.g., overly high discount rates) and illustrate the higher costs associated with private financing. Problems for privatized staff (e.g., lower wages and more precarious working conditions) and privatized support services (e.g., concerns with cleanliness and training), familiar features of P3 projects, are present in all four hospital cases as well.

Aside from issues that tend to occur with all P3s, regardless of the type of project, the three most important concerns unique to P3 hospitals (identified in chapter 2) are also indicated through these four projects. First, their internal bifurcation of authority has made addressing the challenges associated with support-service privatization a time-consuming and frustrating ordeal. Second, local community and third-sector contributions were ratcheted up in response to more expensive capital costs. Third, infrastructure design arrived at in the early 2000s must suffice for the next three decades, reducing policy flexibility and the opportunity to incorporate technological innovations well into the future. Physical alterations in response to future innovation can certainly be made to P3 hospital infrastructure, but this will come at a high cost. As the Diamond Centre example indicates, any changes made to the building must be arranged through the private partner, not the most cost-effective or efficient service-provider; and for this P3 there is also an automatic 15 per cent overhead fee added to the price of any spatial and design reconfiguration.

The higher costs associated with privately financed P3s not only undermine arguments that they help curb wasteful government spending; there is also less available to be spent on other health infrastructure and social concerns. The model also represents a significant departure from a traditional hospital setting where authority and control are fully retained by public sector health authorities, constituting a notable – albeit relatively invisible – restructuring of state and society. Even in the case of hospitals that have been subject to extensive support-service contracting-out, the power sharing inherent to a P3 goes far deeper. With contracting-out, agreements are in place for only a few years at a time rather than several decades, and service contracts are most often kept separate rather than bundled.

Shortly after initiating these pioneering projects, BC and Ontario began to unroll their health sector P3 programs. These programs were launched without actually evaluating the problems and potentials offered by the model, as established through their pioneering P3 hospitals. Instead, proliferation was a foregone conclusion from the start. By creating enabling fields, and the new capital planning frameworks, P3 units, and enabling legislation that allow for the flourishing of P3 programs, policymakers moved the P3 agenda forward in these provincial health sectors in ways that might not have been possible earlier. Enabling fields have normalized the model through features such as the capital planning routines that favour and depoliticize P3 selection, and the creation of P3 units that provide institutional stability and embed the P3 model within public sector decision-making. These efforts have turned the once highly politicized P3 model into the standard way in which hospital projects with a public sector cost in excess of $20/$50 million are delivered in both provinces – effectively making P3s the "new traditional," given that all such projects have since the early 2000s gone forward in this manner.

In both Ontario and BC, P3-enabling fields have helped to greatly improve the appearance of P3 processes by institutionalizing multiple value for money assessment stages, offering protections for the public interest through principles enshrined in capital planning frameworks, standardizing routines and legal documents, and publicizing project information. However, actual improvements in P3 outcomes remain elusive, and thus P3-enabling field improvements are largely artifice. Value for money remains a fundamentally flawed evaluation procedure and continues to employ deceptive methods to help justify privatization,[1] the principles of capital planning frameworks remain toothless (and P3s inherently violate most principles in BC and Ontario), and greater transparency has not translated into the publication of substantially informative project details. The major improvement offered by AFP in Ontario is restricted to items that went far beyond typical practice in BC – bringing contract lengths down from over half a century to three decades, and institutionalizing lease arrangements rather than the full privatization of land and facilities.

Inherent to the entrenchment of P3s has been a reconceptualization of the "public interest." Given that society is class divided, its interests are too, and thus it is no surprise that the "public interest," as represented by public policy, will be as well (Mahon 1977, 170). Health and health care–related concerns remain the key factor in hospital infrastructure design and development, exemplified through an enduring focus on infection control and ensuring reasonable access to health services. Yet these concerns are now subsumed within the matrix of market-based logics and market-like calculus: hospitals leave the proposal stage only

---

1 To reiterate, value for money methodology is biased for several reasons: discount rates are often far too high; risk is double-counted, to the detriment of the public sector comparator (and it is assumed that a PSC cannot transfer risk); risk matrices remain unjustified; uncertainties and risks created by P3s are ignored; and P3 value for money cannot be truly ascertained until after the project agreement expires (which will not happen in any Canadian provincial health sector for decades to come).

when they deliver value for money through the transfer of commer-cially bearable risk. Transferring risk can potentially benefit the wider public interest by helping to keep costs down, thereby improving the long-run sustainability of the public health care system, given that hospitals are a leading cost pressure within the system. However, the myopic focus on certain risks – risks that can generate profit for private partners – ignores other aspects of the public interest such as long-run uncertainties, policy inflexibility, bifurcated hospital decision-making, pressures added to health sector charities and auxiliaries, and an erosion of working conditions for staff, service quality, democratic con-trol, accountability, and transparency. The "public interest" is therefore reconceptualized for the benefit of privatization-enabling concerns, and all other interests are made to fit within that prism. Trade-offs are made, most often to the detriment of broader social concerns.

An important part of this process has been the creation of a new layer of unequal representation (Mahon 1977): the P3 unit that now makes decisions for all ministries on the basis of P3-biased value for money methodology. It should be noted, however, that there are certain varia-tions between these two provinces in how P3 units have been institu-tionalized. Whereas Infrastructure Ontario is largely a creature of the Ministry of Infrastructure and is assigned work by ministries seeking to build capital projects, Partnerships BC is more independent from gov-ernment, though it ultimately reports to the Ministry of Finance, and it charges work fees to its public sector clients. In both provinces, capital planning frameworks dictate that P3s must be considered for all large capital projects, and thus the inclusion of P3 unit decision-making in other ministries' processes is mandatory in each jurisdiction.

Financial Crisis and Policy Stabilization

Longstanding problems associated with P3s were compounded by the 2008 global financial crisis. Financial market volatility led to project delays, renegotiations, and collapsed deals in many sectors, and this affected P3 hospitals that had yet to reach financial close (Mackenzie 2009). By the onset of the 2008 financial crisis, the four pioneering P3 hospitals in Ontario and BC had already entered the relatively low-risk operational phase of their agreements, and thus none of these projects were adversely affected. Despite serious cost pressures imposed by the global financial crisis and ensuing credit crunch, BC and Ontario continued to initiate new P3 hospital deals throughout the crisis. With the onset of a new round of fiscal austerity in several Canadian jurisdictions in 2011/12, one might reasonably expect that the P3 model would be scrapped in favour of lower-cost public procurement. Instead, as has been the case since rebounding in 2010, the model is flourishing once again. A crisis of faith was therefore adverted and the P3 model stabilized.

That the attractiveness of P3s suffered only minor setbacks makes little sense from a strict value for money perspective. The stabilization of P3 policy indicates that at base this form of "alternative service delivery" has always been ideologically driven – not an inherently superior procurement model. In fact, as discussed in the previous section, the reality of P3s is such that instead of offering better value for money, from a long-run perspective their use may hinder the overall sustainability of the public health care system, since P3 hospitals are more costly than the public option, service quality is poorer, innovation is stifled through inflexible decades-long contracts, the use of private financing exposes public health care to crisis-prone global financial markets, and hospital service planning suffers from disintegration. Long-term commitments made to more expensive hospital infrastructure can also create a serious debt overhang, producing cost pressures that may lead to service cuts in other areas, given the rigid nature of P3 contracts. P3 use shows little sign of abating in Canada, the result in large part of the cushioning and institutionalizing effects of enabling fields.

The tenacity of enabling field support holds important implications for the future of neoliberalism, as it embeds within the public sector the marketized logics of accumulation through dispossession and financialization. By entrenching these features, neoliberalism is intensified. There are two key aspects to the role that P3s play in this process: the locking-in of accumulation by dispossession and the promotion of financialization.

First, lock-in: P3s help entrench neoliberalism through decades-long, legally binding contracts. Most project agreements last for thirty years or more, which is an extremely long period, when compared with contracting-out, which typically lasts for only a few years at a time. Of course governments do have the option of rescinding P3 agreements, but in light of other important features of neoliberal lock-in (e.g., trade agreements like NAFTA that protect the rights of foreign investors through binding arbitration), this may be far too costly an option for most governments to consider.

A related issue is the contract bundling that is a core feature of the P3 model, meaning that no one element of the project can be severed from the agreement on the basis of poor performance or a change in government ideology. This makes it extremely difficult/costly to renegotiate P3 contracts, given that all components (e.g., infrastructure, support services, land agreements) are legally bound together (Shrybman 2007, 200). This feature would also make it difficult, though never impossible, for a normative or ideological shift to sweep away any one undesirable component of an existing P3.

Second, P3s are a microcosm of the larger neoliberal accumulation strategy: P3s support and benefit from neoliberal financialization, given that the private finance portion is typically linked to international bond markets and involves large institutional investors such as pension funds or multinational banks/financial institutions, along with being a form of accumulation by dispossession. Thus P3s rely upon normative commitments to neoliberalism while simultaneously normalizing neoliberal rule with each new partnership agreement. Further, the private financing of public infrastructure through P3 schemes encourages a host of other unseemly activities that could generate (unforeseen) problems in the future. Key among these are the promotion of off-balance-sheet accounting practices, the conversion of public goods into private assets that may be repackaged and resold through secondary, often offshore, financial markets with risks ultimately backed by the taxpayer, the commercial confidentiality rules that obscure public and private partner accountability, and profiteering from public infrastructure through refinancing and equity sales (see Reynolds 2011; Sandborn 2008; Whitfield 2009). In sum, efforts to support and promote P3s not only are expressions of neoliberal policy but also help to reinforce its practice and discourse.

Alternatives (and Their Limits)

The entrenchment of P3 policy proceeds not only through the nature of these contracts but also through the normalization of privatization. Depoliticization occurs when authority and decision-making in areas of social concern (such as health care and health services) are shifted away from government and into the private sector. With P3s this happens through the awarding of multi-decade contracts to the for-profit managers who operate these projects, as well as through the private consultants, transaction advisors, accountants, and auditors who come to inform P3 policy. Colin Hay (2007, 80–7) also suggests that depoliticization can occur when social issues are demoted from the government sphere to the public sphere. P3s conform to this type of depoliticization when they shift public infrastructure and service decisions out of the formal democratic arena (where decision-makers are accountable and public deliberation takes place) into the far less transparent realm of arm's-length public sector managers. In BC and Ontario, this role is dominated by P3 units, the quasi-public sector agencies created to promote and evaluate P3s.

Structured as semi-autonomous Crown corporations, Partnerships BC and Infrastructure Ontario are relatively insulated from public accountability, and their decision-making reflects private sector rationales (such as market-oriented value for money and risk transfer). The historical relationship between Canadian Crown corporations and capital has always been less black and white than privatization promoters may suggest – state-owned enterprises do not always crowd out private for-profit competitors, displace private markets, or expropriate private assets. Notwithstanding their social obligations, Crown corporations (particularly those that are commercially oriented) have often supported capital by socializing the costs of production (e.g., Ontario Hydro), reducing what Harvey (2001) calls the "socially necessary turnover time" of capital by aiding capital circulation across this vast country (e.g., CN Rail and Air Canada), paying for research and development (e.g., Petro-Canada), and propping up production and demand in rural and remote locations (e.g., Manitoba Telephone Systems) (discussed in Whiteside 2012). Yet for the first time in Canadian history the legal status of the Crown corporation, with its exemption from certain public sector regulations (e.g., relating to employee pay structures), is being used to facilitate ongoing privatization within the public sector. This constitutes a significant neoliberal reinterpretation of the policy advantages offered by a Crown corporation.

Institutionalization through P3 units, along with routinization through new capital planning procedures and depoliticization, present a formidable challenge to effective resistance and the search for alternatives to privatization. Attempts to resist P3s must be aimed at the (re)politicization of public infrastructure and service procurement. This means targeting not only the outcomes of privatization (i.e., dispossession) but also the processes that encourage and support P3 selection (i.e., enabling fields).

Public sector unions and public service advocacy organizations drive resistance to P3s, and while some efforts have been successful, ultimately P3s are proliferating now more than ever. Resistance has produced several important changes in health sector P3 programs over the years, although it has not yet affected *whether* P3s are used but instead *how* they move forward. One of the most significant changes is the 2006 exemption of soft support services (e.g., housekeeping, food, patient portering) from Ontario's hospital P3 deals, and hospitals recently developed in BC have excluded cleaning services. Concerns around debt refinancing have also led to the inclusion of clauses within Ontario's P3 hospital project agreements that stipulate that financial gains reaped through debt refinancing must now be shared with the relevant public hospital board (Loxley 2010, 110). A reversal of some elements of privatization-enabling legislation has also occurred. Most notably, in 2007 the Supreme Court of Canada sided with BC's Hospital Employees' Union, and other health sector unions, in their fight against BC Bill 29-2002 (The Health and Social Services Delivery Improvement Act), which unilaterally rescinded provisions in signed collective agreements and paved the way for unprecedented privatization of health care support staff in the province. This forced changes to similar unconstitutional provisions in P3-related legislation (BC Bill 94-2003, The Health Sector Partnerships Agreement Act) as well.

The need to protect the public must come in other ways as well. In this struggle it is important to keep in mind that many/most enabling-field items are presented as protections for the "public interest." BC's Capital Asset Management Framework (CAMF) and Ontario's Infrastructure Planning, Financing, and Procurement Framework (IPFP) are touted as both improvements made to the way P3s used to be developed and as innovations that proactively address public concern. Yet CAMF and IPFP best-practice principles[2] not only offer misleading protections (in fact P3s violate nearly every principle), they are also toothless – mechanisms have yet to be put in place that would actually guarantee that their principles are upheld.

Legislation in Manitoba offers one way of rectifying this. In 2012 the province took an important step towards expanding protections for the public with its Bill 34 (The Public-Private Partnerships Transparency and Accountability Act), which requires greater public consultation and

---

2 CAMF: sound fiscal management, strong accountability, value for money, protection of the public interest, and competition and transparency; IPFP: the public interest is paramount, value for money must be demonstrated, appropriate public ownership/control must be preserved, accountability must be maintained, and all processes must be fair, transparent, and efficient.

involvement of officials such as the provincial auditor general and fairness monitors. However, as beneficial as fairness monitors and auditors general may be (provincial auditors' reports have thus far proven to be a leading source of support for anti-P3 campaigns), actual progress will remain illusory until the P3 model is scrapped altogether. Victories and initiatives such as those mentioned above help dampen the more deleterious effects of dispossession but they do not entirely counter it, nor do they root out the specific elements of privatization-driven state restructuring that have occurred over the past decade.

Furthermore, auditors' reports are extremely helpful but they amount to little if their findings do not translate into substantial policy change. The campaign to depoliticize P3 use is only as effective as the electorate allows it to be. For many groups and individuals P3s are seen as a highly politicized and ideologically based policy, but this is not necessarily a common perspective – most clearly indicated through relative apathy in the face of P3 proliferation. A greater focus on P3-enabling fields would be useful for opponents, as it helps to uncover the ways in which privatization by stealth proceeds through the support of even more obscure changes being made to public sector decision-making in some jurisdictions. This includes politicizing the institutionalization, routinization, and normalization of the market-based rationale that informs P3 policy and reorients public sector decision-making.

Finally, it is crucial that P3 opponents develop tangible, viable solutions to the problem of financing public infrastructure. All four P3 hospitals examined in this study languished in the proposal stage for years, sometimes decades. These delays were unacceptable and drove the justification for P3s at the local level. It also dampened resistance. If the choice offered to a community is either a new P3 hospital or no new hospital at all, it ought to be no surprise that opposition to privatization has been marginalized. CUPE (2011, 15–16) describes two excellent solutions to the funding dilemma: greater federal support for the costs of public health care infrastructure (e.g., the creation of a federal Public Asset Fund, as proposed by the Canadian Centre for Policy Alternatives), echoing similar demands by the Canadian Healthcare Association and Association of Canadian Academic Healthcare Organizations; and the use of public bonds to finance hospital infrastructure.[3]

---

3 However, greater public sector reliance upon bond markets would certainly bring its own particular challenges and contradictions, in line with financialization of all stripes.

Solutions such as these would ensure that new projects proceed, and that this is accomplished through the most cost-effective (and publicly beneficial) fashion possible.

P3s have for far too long been misleadingly justified as a "build now, pay later" solution fit for times of fiscal restraint. With the recent return of fiscal austerity, the model is poised to make even greater inroads into public service and infrastructure provision, particularly at the municipal/local level, for it bears the greatest burden associated with budget cuts at a time of dwindling revenue. The federal government is also actively encouraging P3 expansion at the local level through the financial and technical support offered by PPP Canada and the P3 Canada Fund – resources that can be accessed only when a project uses the P3 model.

At all levels of government and regardless of sector, P3s do not come cheap. Private financing is more expensive, social costs are greater, and the loss of public control, oversight, and accountability is anti-democratic. The implications of P3 institutionalization will reverberate for decades to come. Passing on higher-cost, lower-quality, riskier, and less innovative infrastructure and service forms to future generations is no solution to meeting the needs of today.

Appendix

Development Timeline for Canada's Pioneering P3 Hospitals

Abbotsford Regional Hospital and Cancer Centre

2001

- **Spring 2001**: NDP approve a new public hospital in Abbotsford
- **August 2001**: Liberals commission PricewaterhouseCoopers to evaluate the P3 option

2002

- **February 2002**: Budget 2002 introduces a "new approach to capital planning" (P3s), but the Abbotsford hospital still appears as a public hospital in the capital plans
- **March 2002**: PricewaterhouseCoopers report released, which finds a cost savings of 1 per cent over thirty years, assumes the cost of the hospital will be $210 million
- **November 2002**: Premier Campbell announces that the new hospital will be a P3

2003

- **January 2003**: request for expression of interest (REOI) issued
- **February 2003**: Budget 2003 reveals that the hospital no longer appears in the government's capital spending plans
- **May 2003**: four short-listed bidders announced
- **September 2003**: request for proposals issued to four short-listed consortia
- **October 2003**: Fraser Health Authority awards a $73 million, five-year contract to Sodexo Canada for housekeeping in the health authority (in force 1 January 2004)
- **November 2003**: only two bidders remain, after other two pull out

2004

- **January 2004**: support services at the Matsqui-Sumas-Abbotsford hospital are contracted-out to Sodexo
- **February 2004**: one bidder remains: Access Health Abbotsford, after the other pulls out
- **March 2004**: Partnerships BC announces it will conduct a value for money assessment by comparing the P3 option to a public sector comparator over a year after the REOI is issued
- **May 2004 to December 2004**: contract negotiation and finalization phase
- **October 2004**: Partnerships BC sets up Abbotsford Regional Hospital and Cancer Centre Inc. to deal with Access Health Abbotsford and to oversee construction
- **December 2004**: project agreement is signed: private partner will design, build, finance, and operate all non-clinical care services at the facility (operational component will run for thirty years, to begin in 2008)
- **December 2004**: site preparation begins

2005

- **February 2005**: the auditor general releases his attestation report on Partnerships BC's value for money calculations
- **March 2005**: start of construction of foundations

2008

- **April 2008**: substantial completion of construction
- **August 2008**: 121 patients are moved from the Matsqui-Sumas-Abbotsford Hospital to the new Abbotsford Regional Hospital and Cancer Care Centre
- **September 2008**: the hospital opens to new patients
- **September 2008**: the Abbotsford cleaners and food workers vote unanimously in favour of joining the Hospital Employees' Union

Gordon and Leslie Diamond Health Care Centre

2001

- **2001**: site redevelopment approved by the City of Vancouver

2002

- **May 2002**: business case is finalized by the Vancouver Coastal Health Authority, which concludes that a P3 would be most cost-effective approach
- **July 2002**: the province approves plans to deliver the project as a P3 (at this time it is known as the Academic Ambulatory Care Facility)

- **October 2002:** Premier Campbell publicly announces that a P3 will be used
- **October 2002:** the request for expression of interest (REOI) is issued (nine proponents submit responses)

2003
- **April 2003:** three bidders shortlisted
- **June 2003:** the request for proposals (RFP) is issued (two are invited to submit bids, both sent in bids)

2004
- **January 2004:** preferred proponent selected, and negotiation with the preferred bidder begins (the Vancouver Coastal Health Authority refuses to publicly name the preferred bidder)
- **January 2004 to September 2004:** contract negotiation and finalization phase
- **September 2004:** project agreement is signed: private partner will design, build, finance, and operate all non-clinical care services at the facility (operational component will run for thirty years, to begin in 2006)
- **September 2004:** site preparation begins
- **November 2004:** Partnerships BC releases to the public a value for money report

2006
- **June 2006:** Vancouver philanthropists Gordon and Leslie Diamond donate $20 million (not related to P3 financing)
- **October 2006:** Premier Campbell officially opens the Diamond Centre

2007
- **January 2007:** Shoppers Drug Mart opens on the main level

Brampton Civic Hospital

1971
- **1971:** the Chinguacousy County Council votes to spend $300,000 of public money to buy twenty hectares at the northeast corner of Bramalea Road and Bovaird Drive, and passes a bylaw restricting its use to building a public hospital

1997
- **1997:** the Hospital Services Restructuring Committee (HSRC) recommends the amalgamation of Peel Memorial Hospital with Georgetown and District Memorial Hospital and Etobicoke General Hospital; in 1998 these three come

under the administration of the newly created Northwest GTA Hospital Corporation, later renamed the William Osler Health Centre (WOHC), while the HSRC also reaffirms the need for a new hospital in the Brampton region and suggests that Peel Memorial should also be renovated and redeveloped

2000
- **Spring 2000**: the PC government earmarks funds for a new hospital in Brampton. The facility will be the first new hospital built in the area in 30 years

2001
- **November 2001**: Tony Clement (then Minister of Health) and Jim Flaherty (then Minister of Finance and the minister responsible for SuperBuild) announce that the new Brampton hospital will be a P3

2002
- **March 2002**: the Request for Expression of Interest (REOI) is issued. (The REOI asks for bidders to state their interest in contracting for some or all of the work necessary to design, build, finance, own/lease and maintain the health care facility.)
- **May 2002**: the Request for Qualifications (RFQ) is issued (which stipulates that the agreement will involve components relating to designing, building, financing, operating, and managing the facility)
- **July 2002**: groundbreaking ceremony is held to launch the early site preparation works (e.g., major earthworks, connections to sewage and water systems, creation of a storm water retention facility)
- **December 2002**: Ontario Cabinet approves the use of a P3 for the Brampton hospital

2003
- **January 2003**: the hospital board (William Osler Health Centre, WOHC) produces its initial estimate of what the hospital would cost if a traditional public approach was used, almost a year after the REOI was issued
- **April 2003**: the preferred bidder is selected and contract negotiation begin
- **Spring/summer 2003**: Dalton McGuinty, Liberal party leader, vows to dismantle plans to develop the Brampton hospital as a P3
- **September 2003**: a coalition of labour unions and public health care advocates (CUPE, the Ontario Public Service Employees Union, and the Ontario Health Coalition) launch a court action to stop the signing of the P3 deal
- **October 2003**: the Ontario general provincial election is held, in which Liberals win seventy-two seats, PCs twenty-four, NDP seven

- **October 2003**: the coalition of unions and public health care advocates lose their court case on the grounds that there was insufficient evidence to back their claim that P3 hospitals contravene the Public Hospitals Act and Canada Health Act
- **November 2003**: newly appointed Liberal health minister George Smitherman announces that the Brampton hospital project will proceed but the P3 plan will be renegotiated (according to Smitherman, the biggest difference with the Liberal version is that the public will now pay a "mortgage" and fully own the facility once the project agreement expire, while under the PC plan, the facility would have been a lease-to-own agreement with the land and facility privately owned for the length of the project agreement)
- **November 2003 to November 2004**: contract renegotiation and finalization phase

2004
- **November 2004**: financial close is reached on the project
- **November 2004**: WOHC updates its estimate of what the hospital would cost if a traditional public approach was used, after negotiations with the preferred bidder had concluded
- **November 2004**: the project agreement is finalized and The Healthcare Infrastructure Company of Canada (THICC) is chosen to design, build, and finance the new hospital; the twenty-five-year non-clinical-care support service contract begins in October 2007
- **November 2004**: construction begins

2007
- **July 2007**: construction is completed and the hospital officially opens
- **October 2007**: patients are transferred from Peel Memorial Hospital to Brampton Civic Hospital
- **October 2007**: Brampton Civic Hospital begins admitting new patients

Royal Ottawa Hospital

1995

- **1995**: non-clinical care services are contracted out at the Royal Ottawa Hospital

1997
- **February 1997**: the Health Services Restructuring Commissions (HSRC) announces that the Brockville Psychiatric Hospital will be closed down within two years and 140 patients will be moved to the Royal Ottawa Hospital

1999

- **1999**: the hospital board initiates redevelopment plans for the facility

2000

- **May 2000**: ROHCC announces that negotiations have begun with the provincial government to demolish the facility and replace it with a new hospital (guided by the SuperBuild capital planning framework)

2001

- **May 2001**: the PC government announces that P3s would have to be first considered before the government would commit to funding any new hospitals
- **November 2001**: Tony Clement (minister of health) and Jim Flaherty (minister of finance and the minister responsible for SuperBuild) announce that the new Royal Ottawa hospital will be a P3
- **December 2001:** the plans to develop the Royal Ottawa Hospital as a P3 are formally approved by Cabinet

2002

- **June 2002**: the request for qualifications phase begins
- **September 2002**: the hospital board announces that the request for qualifications has produced three shortlisted candidates
- **December 2002**: the request for proposals stage begins

2003

- **May 2003**: negotiations begin with the preferred bidder
- **Spring/summer 2003**: Dalton McGuinty, Liberal party leader, vows to dismantle plans to develop the Royal Ottawa Hospital as a P3
- **September 2003**: a coalition of labour unions and public health care advocates (CUPE, the Ontario Public Service Employees Union, and the Ontario Health Coalition) launch a court action to stop the signing of the P3 deal
- **September 2003**: mere days before the election is held, ROHCC is reported to have finalized the P3 agreement with the preferred proponent, but the agreement had yet to reach commercial and financial close, and after the election, Liberals made several changes to the project agreement (ensuring public ownership of the land and facility)
- **October 2003**: the Ontario general provincial election is held, in which Liberals win seventy-two seats, PCs twenty-four, NDP seven
- **October 2003**: the coalition of unions and public health care advocates lose their court case on the grounds that there was insufficient evidence to back their claim that P3 hospitals contravene the Public Hospitals Act and Canada Health Act

2004

- **July 2004**: renegotiations with the preferred partner conclude (commercial close is achieved)
- **July 2004**: the Royal Ottawa Hospital project agreement is signed as a twenty-one-year design, build, finance, operate and maintain P3 with The Health Infrastructure Company of Canada (THICC); however, alterations made under the McGuinty Liberals include a reduction in the length of the operational phase of the P3 (from what would have likely been sixty-six years), and amendments made to the legal arrangements relating to the ownership of the land and facility (similar to the Brampton hospital)
- **December 2004**: financial close is reached
- **December 2004**: construction begins

2006

- **October 2006**: official opening of the Royal Ottawa Hospital
- **November 2006**: patients are transferred into the new facility

References

"Accountability Is Missing from the Community Charter." 2003. *Vancouver Sun*, 14 March.

Adam, M. 2003. "Liberals Will Let ROH Expansion 'Go Ahead.'" *Ottawa Citizen*, 28 May.

–. 2004. "Liberals Are Hiding ROH Deal, NDP Says: New Pact Same as the Old One, Official Says." *Ottawa Citizen*, 9 January.

–. 2008. "Chronic Complaint." *Ottawa Citizen*, 24 February.

–. 2009. "Audit on Royal Ottawa Sought; Same Group That Built Centre Blasted by Auditor over Brampton Hospital Costs." *Ottawa Citizen*, 26 January.

Aglietta, M. 1998. "Capitalism at the Turn of the Century: Regulation Theory and the Challenge of Social Change." *New Left Review* 232:41–90.

Akintoye, A., M. Beck, and C. Hardcastle, eds. 2003. *Public-Private Partnerships: Managing Risks and Opportunities*. Oxford: Blackwell. http://dx.doi.org/10.1002/9780470690703.

Alleyne, R. 2012. "Six Other NHS Trusts at Risk of 'Bankruptcy.'" *Telegraph*, 26 June. http://www.telegraph.co.uk/news/health/news/9356064/Six-other-NHS-trusts-at-risk-of-bankruptcy.html.

Anderson, J. 2008. "Cities Debate Privatizing Public Infrastructure." *New York Times*, 26 August. http://www.nytimes.com.

Armitstead, L. 2012. "UK Taxpayers 'Rarely' Benefit from Public-Private Partnerships, Claims Study." *Telegraph*, 11 April. http://www.telegraph.co.uk/finance/newsbysector/constructionandproperty/9196524/UK-taxpayers-rarely-benefit-from-public-private-partnerships-claims-study.html.

Armstrong, H. 1977. "The Labour Force and State Workers in Canada." In *The Canadian State: Political Economy and Political Power*, ed. Leo Panitch, 289–310. Toronto: University of Toronto Press.

Armstrong, P., and H. Armstrong. 2008. *Health Care*. Halifax: Fernwood.
–. 2010. "Contradictions at Work: Struggles for Control in Canadian Health Care." *Socialist Register* 46:145–67.
Arrighi, G., N. Aschoff, and B. Scully. 2010. "Accumulation by Dispossession and Its Limits: The South Africa Paradigm Revisited." *Studies in Comparative International Development* 45 (4): 410–38. http://dx.doi.org/10.1007/s12116-010-9075-7.
Ascoli, U., and C. Ranci. 2002. "The Context of New Social Policies in Europe." In *Dilemmas of the Welfare Mix*, ed. U. Ascoli and C. Ranci, 1–24. New York: Kluwer. http://dx.doi.org/10.1007/978-1-4757-4992-2_1.
Ashman, S., and A. Callinicos. 2006. "Capital Accumulation and the State System: Assessing David Harvey's *The New Imperialism*." *Historical Materialism* 14 (4): 107–31. http://dx.doi.org/10.1163/156920606778982572.
"Audit on Royal Ottawa Sought." 2009. *Ottawa Citizen*, 26 January. http://ottawacitizen.com.
Auditor General. 2011. *Audit of the Academic Ambulatory Care Centre Public Private Partnership: Vancouver Coastal Health Authority*. May. Victoria, BC: Office of the Auditor General. http://www.bcauditor.com/pubs/2011/report2/public-private-partnership-P3-audit-VCHA-AACC.
–. 2012. *Audits of the Two P3 Projects in the Sea-to-Sky Corridor*. July. Victoria, BC: Office of the Auditor General. http://www.bcauditor.com/pubs/2012/report4/audits-two-p3-projects-sea-sky-corridor.
Auerbach, L., A. Donner, D.D. Peters, M. Townson, and A. Yalnizyan. 2003. *Funding Hospital Infrastructure: Why P3s Don't Work, and What Will*. Ottawa: Canadian Centre for Policy Alternatives. http://www.policyalternatives.ca/sites/default/files/uploads/publications/National_Office_Pubs/p3_hospitals.pdf.
Bailey, I. 2012. "BC Appoints Municipal Auditor-General." *Globe and Mail*, 7 November. http://www.theglobeandmail.com/news/british-columbia/bc-appoints-municipal-auditor-general/article5069238/.
Ball, R., M. Heafy, and D. King. 2001. "The Private Finance Initiative: A Good Deal for the Public Purse or a Drain on Future Generations?" *Policy and Politics* 29 (1): 95–108. http://dx.doi.org/10.1332/0305573012501224.
Barker, P. 1986. "Hospital Promised by Premier a Political Hot Potato." *Toronto Star*, 28 October.
Barlow, J., and M. Köberle-Gaiser. 2008. "The Private Finance Initiative, project form and design innovation: The UK's hospital programme." *Research Policy* 37 (8): 1392–402.
Barrett, M., and M. Hodnett. 2010. "MOHLTC/LHIN Joint Review Framework for Early Capital Planning Stages." Presented to Ministry and LHIN Staff by CEO

of South West LHIN and manager of GTA Capital Team, Health Capital Investment Branch, MOHLTC, 28 October. http://www.centraleastlhin.on.ca.

"BC Health Authorities Cut Costs to Meet Budgets." 2009. CBC News, 15 July. http://www.cbc.ca/news/canada/british-columbia/b-c-health-authorities-cut-costs-to-meet-budgets-1.835915.

BC Liberal Party. 2009. "The Real Story ... on the NDP and Public-Private Partnerships." April. http://www.bcliberals.com.

BC Ministry of Community Services. 2005. *Introduction to Regional Districts: Communities in Partnership*. http://www.fvrd.bc.ca/Documents/Regional%20District%20Toolkit%20-%20Booklet%20-%20Intro%20to%20RD%27s.pdf.

BC Ministry of Finance. n.d. "Overview." *Capital Asset Management Framework*. http://www.fin.gov.bc.ca/tbs/camf_overview.pdf.

–. 2002. "New Framework, Agency to Guide Public Building." News release, 30 May.

–. 2008. "Province Raises Capital Standard Threshold for PPPs." News release, 7 November. http://www2.news.gov.bc.ca/news_releases_2005-2009/2008FIN0019-001677.htm.

BC Ministry of Health Planning. 2002. *A New Era for Patient-Centred Health Care*. www.health.gov.bc.ca/socsec/pdf/new_era_sustain.pdf.

BC Ministry of Health Services. 2003. *Report on Health Authority Performance Agreements 2002/03*. http://www.health.gov.bc.ca/socsec/pdf/haagreement0203.pdf.

BC Ministry of Municipal Affairs. 1999. *Public Private Partnership: A Guide for Local Government*. May. http://www.cscd.gov.bc.ca/lgd/policy_research/library/public_private_partnerships.pdf.

BC Nurses Union (BCNU). 2003. "Bill Reveals Private Firm Will Own New Abbotsford Hospital." News release, 20 November.

BC Office of the Premier. 2012. "Premier Announces First Auditor General for Local Government." News release, 7 November. http://www2.news.gov.bc.ca/news_releases_2009-2013/2012PREM0137-001734.htm.

BC Select Standing Committee on Public Accounts. 2006. "Auditor General Review of Partnership B.C. Report: *Achieving Value for Money: Abbotsford Regional Hospital and Cancer Centre Project*." 8 February. http://www.leg.bc.ca/cmt/38thparl/session-1/pac/hansard/p60208a.htm#6:1245.

–. 2011. *Auditor General Report: Audit of the Academic Ambulatory Care Centre Public Private Partnership: Vancouver Coastal Health Authority*. 27 June. http://www.leg.bc.ca/cmt/39thparl/session-3/pac/hansard/P10627a.htm#17:1155.

Berger, P., J. Tyson, I. Karpowicz, and M. Delgado Coelho. 2009. "The Effects of the Financial Crisis on Public-Private Partnerships." IMF Working Paper. IMF Fiscal Affairs Department. July.

Bezanson, K., and M. Luxton. 2006. "Social Reproduction and Feminist Political Economy." In *Rethinking Social Reproduction: Feminist Political Economy Challenges Neo-Liberalism*, ed. K. Bezanson and M. Luxton, 3–10. Montreal and Kingston: McGill-Queen's University Press.

Bish, R.L. 1990. *Local Government in British Columbia*. 2nd ed. Richmond, BC: Union of British Columbia Municipalities.

Bish, R.L., and E.G. Clemens. 2008. *Local Government in British Columbia*. 4th ed. Richmond, BC: Union of British Columbia Municipalities.

Blackwell, T. 2003. "Liberals Vow to Reverse Private Hospital Move." *National Post*, 23 May.

Block, S. 2008. *From P3s to AFP*. Canadian Centre for Policy Alternatives. May. http://www.policyalternatives.ca/sites/default/files/uploads/publications/Ontario_Office_Pubs/2008/From_P3s_to_AFPs.pdf.

Boyer, R., and Y. Saillard, eds. 1995. *Regulation Theory*. New York: Routledge.

Boyle, T. 2001. "Ontario Wooing Hospital Landlords, Plans to Open Door to Private Construction, Ownership." *Toronto Star*, 1 December.

Boyne, G.A. 1998. *Public Choice Theory and Local Government: A Comparative Analysis of the UK and the USA*. Basingstoke, UK: Macmillan. http://dx.doi.org/10.1057/9780230373099.

Brenner, R. 2006. "What Is, and What Is Not, Imperialism?" *Historical Materialism* 14 (4): 79–105. http://dx.doi.org/10.1163/156920606778982464.

Broadbent, J., J. Gill, and R. Laughlin. 2003. "Evaluating the Private Finance Initiative in the National Health Service in the UK." *Accounting, Auditing & Accountability Journal* 16 (3): 422–45. http://dx.doi.org/10.1108/09513570310482309.

Burnham, P. 2001. "New Labour and the Politics of Depoliticization." *British Journal of Politics and International Relations* 3 (2): 127–49. http://dx.doi.org/10.1111/1467-856X.00054.

Campbell, R. 2006. "Doctor Executive Earns Leadership Honours." *Medical Post* 42 (26), 22 August.

"Campbell Dodged Questions." 2002. *Maple Ridge, Pitt Meadows Times*, 25 October.

"Canada: An Intelligence Report." 2010. *Infrastructure Investor*. December/January. http://www.p3canada.ca/~/media/english/resources-library/files/other%20canada%20an%20intelligence%20report.pdf.

Canadian Council for Public-Private Partnerships (CCPPP). n.d. "Definitions." http://www.pppcouncil.ca/resources/about-ppp/definitions.html.

–. 2005. "Ontario Infrastructure Minister Announces New Infrastructure Agency & Financing Method." *For the Record*. May. http://www.pppcouncil.ca/pdf/caplanftr2.pdf.

–. 2009. *The Impact of Global Credit Retraction on the Canadian PPP Market*. Toronto: Canadian Council for Public-Private Partnerships.

Canadian Institute for Health Information (CIHI). 2012. *National Health Expenditure Trends, 1975–2012*. Ottawa: Canadian Institute for Health Information.

Canadian Labour Congress (CLC). 2009. "Budget 2009: Economic Crisis, P3s and Municipalities." Canadian Labour Congress. 13 March. http://www.congresdutravail.ca/sites/default/files/pdfs/2009-03-13-Budget_and_Municipalities_0.pdf

Canadian Union of Public Employees (CUPE). 1998. Behind the Pretty Packaging: Exposing Public-Private Partnerships. Ottawa: CUPE.

–. 2003. "Exposing PPPs." http://cupe.ca/privatization.

–. 2009. "Quebec Government Backs Away from P3s." 23 June. http://cupe.ca/privatization.

–. 2011. *P3 Hospitals: The Wrong Direction*. http://cupe.ca/privatization.

Capital Project Plan. Academic Ambulatory Care Centre. (CPP AACC). 2004. "Capital Project Plan. Academic Ambulatory Care Centre." *Budget Transparency and Accountability Act: Disclosure*. October. http://www.partnershipsbc.ca/pdf/AACC_BTAA_report_Final_Oct2704.pdf.

Cayo, D. 2005. "Only One Bid Received to Build, Run BC's Second Big P3 Deal." *Vancouver Sun*, 23 February.

Clarke, D. 2010. "Health Capital Investment in Ontario." Paper presented to Design & Health Canada, 7 June. http://www.designandhealth.com/uploaded/documents/International-Symposium/Canada/Presentations/David-Clarke.pdf.

Clarke, J. 2008. "Living with/in and without Neo-liberalism." *Focaal: European Journal of Anthropology* 2008 (51): 135–47.

Cohen, M.G., and M. Cohen. 2006. "Privatization: A Strategy for Eliminating Pay Equity in Health Care." In *Social Reproduction: Feminist Political Economy Challenges Neo-Liberalism*, ed. K. Bezanson and M. Luxton, 117–44. Montreal and Kingston: McGill-Queen's University Press.

Cohn, D. 2004. "The Public-Private Partnership 'Fetish': Moving beyond the Rhetoric." *Revue Gouvernance* 1 (2): 1–24.

–. 2006. "Transformative Change and Measuring Success: Public-Private Partnerships in British Columbia, 2001–2005." *Revue Gouvernance* 3 (2): 1–21.

–. 2008. "British Columbia's Capital Asset Management Framework: Moving from a Transactional to Transformative Leadership on Public-Private Partnerships, or a 'Railroad Job'?" *Canadian Public Administration* 51 (1): 71–97. http://dx.doi.org/10.1111/j.1754-7121.2008.00005.x.

Colverson, S. 2012. *Harnessing the Power of Public-Private Partnerships: The Role of Hybrid Financing Strategies in Sustainable Development*. International

Institute for Sustainable Development. http://www.iisd.org/pdf/2012/harnessing_ppp.pdf.

"Construction Completed for William Osler Health Centre's Brampton Civic Hospital: On Time, on Budget and Scheduled to Open to Patients October 28, 2007." 2007. Canada News Wire, 3 July.

Cox, R.W, with T.J. Sinclair. 1996. *Approaches to World Order*. Cambridge: Cambridge University Press. http://dx.doi.org/10.1017/CBO9780511607905.

Deloitte Consulting. 2000. *Capital Management Process Review for the Government of British Columbia: Final Report*. April.

Denley, R. 2000. "ROH Wants Brand-New, $85-Million Facility: Officials Asking Province for OK to Replace Current Buildings." *Ottawa Citizen*, 13 May.

Depner, W. 2002. "Community Charter Would Give City Council Power Plus." *Penticton Western* 36 (25), 30 March. http://www.fonvca.org/Issues/Community-Charter/Penticton-Western-30mar02.pdf.

Dix, A. 2003. "Private Hospital Plan Brings High Costs." *Times Colonist*, 3 November.

Drapak, F. 2009. "How the Financial Crisis Has Changed the Market for PPPs: Presentation Transcript." World Bank Institute.

"Dubious Financing for Health Facility." 2005. *Toronto Star*, 17 September.

Dunsky, I., and L. Stougiannos. 2013. "Canada: The Success of P3 in Canada." Mondaq. http://www.mondaq.com/canada/x/256856/Government+Contracts+Procurement+PPP/The+Success+of+P3+in+Canada.

Dutz, M., C. Harris, I. Dhingra, and C. Shugart. 2006. *Public-Private Partnership Units*. World Bank.

Dyer, T. 1987. "Psychiatric Wards Are so Full Patients Sent Home during Night." *Toronto Star*, 27 May 27.

Edwards, P., and J. Shaoul. 2003. "Partnerships: For Better or Worse?" *Accounting, Auditing & Accountability Journal* 16 (3): 397–421. http://dx.doi.org/10.1108/09513570310482345.

Egan, K. 2001. "New Royal Ottawa Will Promote 'Healing' and 'Hope': An 'Enlightened' Public-Private Partnership Will Be the Wave of the Future in Health Care, Say Provincial Politicians." *Ottawa Citizen*, 8 December.

Enchin, H. 2002. "Campbell Keen to Pursue P3s 'That Work.'" *Vancouver Sun*, 5 June.

Evans, M.B., and J. Shields. 1998. *"Reinventing" the Third Sector: Alternative Service Delivery, Partnerships and the New Public Administration of the Canadian Post-Welfare State*. Centre for Voluntary Sector Studies. Faculty of Business. Ryerson University. Working Paper Series, no. 9. May.

–. 2000. *Neoliberal Restructuring and the Third Sector: Reshaping Governance, Civil Society and Local Relations*. Centre for Voluntary Sector Studies.

Faculty of Business. Ryerson University. Working Paper Series, no. 13. July.

Evans, R.G. 2008. "The World Is Not the Way They Tell You It Is." Introductory lecture, Executive MBA Program, Sauder School, University of British Columbia. Centre for Health Services and Policy Research, University of British Columbia. 4 April.

Farnsworth, K. 2006. "Capital to the Rescue? New Labour's Business Solutions to Old Welfare Problems." *Critical Social Policy* 26 (4): 817–42.

Farquharson, E., and J. Encinas. 2010. "The UK Treasury Infrastructure Finance Unit: Supporting PPPs Financing during the Global Liquidity Crisis." *Public-Private Partnerships Solutions*. World Bank Institute. March. http://siteresources.worldbank.org/WBI/Resources/213798-1259011531325/6598384-1268250365374/PPP_Solutions_01.pdf.

Farrugia, C., T. Reynolds, and R.J. Orr. 2008. *Public-Private Partnership Agencies: A Global Perspective*. Collaboratory for Research on Global Projects, Stanford University. Working paper no. 39. August. http://www.nawc.org/uploads/documents-and-publications/documents/document_02445830-0b21-4f61-8b65-bad5f5989467.pdf.

Fawcett, G. 2012. "Public Private Partnerships: The Record Isn't Great." *Guardian*, 11 April. http://www.theguardian.com/public-leaders-network/blog/2012/apr/11/public-private-partnerships-the-record-isnt-great.

Ferguson, J. 1995. *The Anti-Politics Machine: "Development," Depoliticization and Bureaucratic Power in Lesotho*. Minneapolis: University of Minnesota Press.

Fine, B. 2006. "Debating the 'New' Imperialism." *Historical Materialism* 14 (4): 133–56. http://dx.doi.org/10.1163/156920606778982536.

Fine, B., and D. Hall. 2012. "Terrains of Neoliberalism." In *Alternatives to Privatization*, ed. D.A. MacDonald and G. Ruiters, 45–70. New York: Routledge.

Finkel, A. 1977. "Origins of the Welfare State in Canada." In Panitch, *Canadian State*, 344–70.

Francis, R. 2006. "Carole Taylor Justifies CEO Larry Blain's Big Salary." *Georgia Straight*, 2 November. http://www.straight.com/news/carole-taylor-justifies-ceo-larry-blains-big-salary.

Fraser Health Authority (FHA). n.d. "Our Board." http://www.fraserhealth.ca/about_us/leadership/board-of-directors/board_members/.

–. 2009. *Service Plan, 2009/10–2011/12*. http://www.fraserhealth.ca/media/ServicePlan09.pdf.

–. 2011. *Service Plan, 2011/12–2013/14*. http://www.fraserhealth.ca/media/ServicePlan%20_2011.pdf.

Fraser, I. 2009. "John Swinney Slams PFI Legacy." *Sunday Times*, 19 April. http://www.thesundaytimes.co.uk/sto.

Fraser Valley Regional District (FVRD). n.d. "Fraser Valley Regional Hospital District." http://www.fvrd.bc.ca/INSIDETHEFVRD/DEPARTMENTS/FINANCE/Pages/FraserValleyRegionalHospitalDistrict.aspx.

Freedland, M. 1998. "Public Law and Private Finance: Placing the Private Finance Initiative in a Public Law Frame." *Public Law* 49 (2) 288–307.

Friedman, M. 1962. *Capitalism and Freedom*. Chicago: University of Chicago Press.

Froud, J. 2003. "The Private Finance Initiative: Risk, Uncertainty and the State." *Accounting, Organizations and Society* 28 (6): 567–89. http://dx.doi.org/10.1016/S0361-3682(02)00011-9.

Fuller, C. 1998. *Caring for Profit*. Ottawa: Canadian Centre for Policy Alternatives.

Funston, M. 1991. "City Needs Hospital Major to Tell Rae." *Toronto Star*, 5 December.

Gaffney, D., A.M. Pollock, D. Price, and J. Shaoul. 1999. "PFI in the NHS: Is There an Economic Case?" *British Medical Journal* 319 (7202): 116–19. http://dx.doi.org/10.1136/bmj.319.7202.116.

Goldsworthy, R. 2002. "Objective Based Government Remains Liberal Target in BC." *Journal of Commerce* 91 & 92, November.

Gordon, M. 1981. *Government in Business*. Montreal: CD Howe.

Government of Canada. 2012. "Budget Plan: Jobs, Growth and Long-term Prosperity – Economic Action Plan 2012." http://www.budget.gc.ca/2012/home-accueil-eng.html.

–. 2013. "The New Building Canada Plan." Budget 2013. http://www.fin.gc.ca/new_template/2013/doc/plan/chap3-3-eng.html.

Government of Nova Scotia. 2008. "Projects Selected for Strategic Infrastructure Partnerships: Transportation and Infrastructure Renewal." 31 July. http://novascotia.ca/news/release/?id=20080731002.

Gramsci, A. 1971. *Selections from the Prison Notebooks of Antonio Gramsci*. Ed. and trans. Q. Hoare and G.N. Smith. New York: International Publishers.

Greenaway, J., B. Salter, and S. Hart. 2004. "The Evolution of a 'Meta-Policy': The Case of the Private Finance Initiative and the Health Sector." *British Journal of Politics and International Relations* 6 (4): 507–26.

Grimsey, D., and M.K. Lewis. 2004. *Public Private Partnerships*. Cheltenham, UK: Edward Elgar. http://dx.doi.org/10.4337/9781845423438.

Guest, D. 1980. *The Emergence of Social Security in Canada*. Vancouver: UBC Press.

Harrison, D. 2001. "Gov't May Lease New Hospital from Owner." *Province*, 19 October.

–. 2003. "2 Firms Drop Bids to Operate Services at Planned Hospital." *Province*, 28 November.

Harvey, D. 2001. *Spaces of Capital*. New York: Routledge.

–. 2003. *The New Imperialism*. Oxford: Oxford University Press.

–. 2004. "The 'New' Imperialism: Accumulation by Dispossession." In *Socialist Register 2004*, ed. L. Panitch and C. Leys, 63–87. London: Merlin.

–. 2006. *The Limits to Capital*. 2nd ed. London: Verso.

Hatcher, R. 2006. "Privatization and Sponsorship: The Re-Agenting of the School System in England." *Journal of Education Policy* 21 (5): 599–619. http://dx.doi.org/10.1080/02680930600866199.

Hay, C. 2004. "The Normalizing Role of Rationalist Assumptions in the Institutional Embedding of Neoliberalism." *Economy and Society* 33 (4): 500–27. http://dx.doi.org/10.1080/0308514042000285260.

–. 2007. *Why We Hate Politics*. Cambridge: Polity.

Heald, D., and G. Georgiou. 2010. "Accounting for PPPs in a Converging World." In *International Handbook on Public-Private Partnerships*, ed. G.A. Hodge, C. Greve, and A.E. Boardman, 237–61. Cheltenham, UK: Edward Elgar. http://dx.doi.org/10.4337/9781849804691.00019.

Hellowell, M. 2013. "PFI Redux?: Assessing a New Model for Financing Hospitals." *Health Policy (Amsterdam)* 113 (1–2): 77–85. http://dx.doi.org/10.1016/j.healthpol.2013.09.008.

Hellowell, M., and A. Pollock. 2007. *Private Finance, Public Deficits: A Report on the Cost of PFI and Its Impact on Health Services in England*. Edinburgh: Centre for International Public Health Policy, University of Edinburgh.

Hellowell, M., and V. Vicchi. 2012. "The Credit Crunch in Infrastructure Finance: Assessing the Economic Advantage of Recent Policy Actions." Paper given at the PPPs for Economic Advantage Conference, Copenhagen, 26 August.

Hill, P. 2003. "Official Outlines Three Elements to Establishing P3's: Council for P3's Conference." *Daily Commercial News and Construction Record* 76:227, 28 November.

Hodge, G. 2000. *Privatization: An International Review of Performance*. Boulder, CO: Westview.

–. 2004. "Risks in Public-Private Partnerships: Shifting, Sharing or Shirking?" *Asia Pacific Journal of Public Administration* 26 (2): 155–79. http://dx.doi.org/10.1080/23276665.2004.10779291.

Hodge, G.A., and C.F. Duffield. 2010. "The Australian PPP Experience: Observations and Reflections." In Hodge, Greve, and Boardman, *International Handbook on Public-Private Partnerships*, 399–438.

Hodge, G.A., and C. Greve. 2005. *The Challenge of Public-Private Partnerships: Learning from International Experience*. Cheltenham, UK: Edward Elgar.

Hood, C. 1991. "A Public Management for All Seasons?" *Public Administration* 69 (1): 3–19. http://dx.doi.org/10.1111/j.1467-9299.1991.tb00779.x.

Hope, C. 2012. "PFI Contracts 'Costing Departments 12 Times More Than They Raise.'" *Telegraph*, 16 May. http://www.telegraph.co.uk/news/politics/9270816/PFI-contracts-costing-departments-12-times-more-than-they-raise.html.

Hoser, T., G. Gilbert, and D. Adams. 2012. "A Tale of Two Markets." *P3 Bulletin*, 7 September. http://www.p3bulletin.com/features/view/1111.

Hospital Employees' Union (HEU). 2004a. "MSA Hospital a Blood-Smeared, Filthy Mess under Sodexho: News Report." *HEU Newsletter*, 11 March.

–. 2004b. "Workers' Rights Violated by BC Liberals' Bill 37." April 28. http://www.heu.org/bargaining/bargaining-bulletins/workers%E2%80%99-rights-violated-bc-liberals%E2%80%99-bill-37.

–. 2008. "Government Policy Paved Way for Low Wages for Hospital Cleaners and Dietary Workers." News release, 27 March. http://www.heu.org/news-media/news-releases/government-policy-paved-way-low-wages-hospital-cleaners-and-dietary-workers.

–. 2012. "HEU Calls for Overhaul of Hospital Cleaning Audits." News release, 1 March. http://www.heu.org/sites/default/files/uploads/news/2012/03/01/NR%2003-01-12%20BG%20Cdiff.pdf.

Hunter, J. 2009. "BC Assumes Larger Share of Financing for Twinning of Port Mann Bridge." *Globe and Mail*, 28 January.

Huws, U. 2012. "Crisis as Capitalist Opportunity: The New Accumulation through Public Service Commodification." *Socialist Register* 48:64–84.

Iacobacci, M. 2010. *Dispelling the Myths: A Pan-Canadian Assessment of Public-Private Partnerships for Infrastructure Investments.* Conference Board of Canada. January.

"Infrastructure Bonds: Who Considers Them?" 2012. *NB Bulletin* 15 (3). http://www.normandin-beaudry.ca/publications/communiques/archives/2012/vol15-n3.en.html.

Infrastructure Ontario. n.d. "Major Projects." http://www.infrastructureontario.ca/Templates/Projects.aspx?id=36&langtype=1033.

–. 2007a. *Assessing Value for Money: A Guide to Infrastructure Ontario's Methodology.* Toronto: Queen's Printer. http://www.infrastructureontario.ca/WorkArea/DownloadAsset.aspx?id=2147488713.

–. 2007b. *Value for Money Assessment: North Bay Regional Health Centre.* Toronto: Queen's Printer. http://www.infrastructureontario.ca/WorkArea/DownloadAsset.aspx?id=2147484529.

–. 2007c. *Value for Money Assessment: Sunnybrook Health Science Centre Redevelopment Project.* Toronto: Queen's Printer. http://www.infrastructureontario.ca/What-We-Do/Projects/AFP-Projects.

–. 2010. *Value for Money Assessment: Centre for Addiction and Mental Health*. Toronto: Queen's Printer. http://www.infrastructureontario.ca/What-We-Do/Projects/Project-Profiles/Centre-for-Addiction-and-Mental-Health-(CAMH).

–. 2011. *2010–2011 Annual Report*. Ontario Infrastructure Projects Corporation. http://www.infrastructureontario.ca/WorkArea/DownloadAsset.aspx?id=2147488402.

Infrastructure UK. 2010. *National Infrastructure Plan 2010*. London: HM Treasury.

Interior Health Authority (IHA). 2008. *Health Service Plan, 2008–2011*. British Columbia. http://www.health.gov.bc.ca/socsec/serviceplan.html.

–. 2011. *2011/12–2013/14 Service Plan*. http://www.interiorhealth.ca/AboutUs/Accountability/Documents/Service%20Plan%202011-12_2013-14.pdf.

Jessop, B. 2002. *The Future of the Capitalist State*. Cambridge: Polity.

–. 2010. "The Continuing Ecological Dominance of Neoliberalism in the Crisis." In *Economic Transitions to Neoliberalism in Middle-income Countries*, ed. A. Saad-Filho and G.L. Yalman, 24–38. London: Routledge.

Jessop, B., and N.-L. Sum. 2006. *Beyond the Regulation Approach*. Cheltenham, UK: Edward Elgar. http://dx.doi.org/10.4337/9781845428907.

Jooste, S.F., R.E. Levitt, and W.R. Scott. 2010. "Beyond 'One Size Fits All': How Local Conditions Shape PPP-Enabled Field Development." Paper presented at the Engineering Project Organizations Conference, South Lake Tahoe, CA, 4–7 November.

Jooste, S.F., and W.R. Scott. 2012. "The Public-Private Partnership Enabling Field: Evidence from Three Cases." *Administration & Society* 44 (2): 149–82. http://dx.doi.org/10.1177/0095399711413868.

Keil, R. 2009. "The Urban Politics of Roll-with-It Neoliberalization." *City* 13 (2–3): 230–45. http://dx.doi.org/10.1080/13604810902986848.

Kettl, D.F. 2005. *The Global Public Management Revolution*. 2nd ed. Washington, DC: Brookings Institution.

Keung, N. 2003. "P3 Hospital Violates Old Bylaws, Says Ex-Reeve: County Bought Land for Centre in '71 Plan Leaves Retiree 'Flabbergasted.'" *Toronto Star*, 4 October.

Knappett, J. 2008. "P3s (or 'No Country for Old Contractors')." *Business Examiner*. March. http://www.cupe.bc.ca/sites/default/files/knappett-no-country-old-contractors_0.pdf.

Kotz, D.M. 1994. "Interpreting the Social Structure of Accumulation." In *Social Structure of Accumulation*, ed. D.M. Kotz, T. McDonough, and M. Reich., 50–71. Cambridge: Cambridge University Press.

Laird, D., and G. Langill. 2005. "A Public/Private Partnership: The Royal Ottawa Hospital Experience." *Healthcare Quarterly* 8 (4): 70–9. http://dx.doi.org/10.12927/hcq..17695.

Larner, W. 2000. "Neoliberalism: Policy, Ideology, Governmentality." *Studies in Political Economy* 63:5–25.

Leigland, J., and Russell, H. 2009. "Another Lost Decade? Effects of the Financial Crisis on Project Finance for Infrastructure." *Gridlines, Public-Private Infrastructure Advisory Facility* 48:1–4.

Leiringer, R. 2006. "Technological Innovation in PPPs: Incentives, Opportunities and Actions." *Construction Management and Economics* 24 (3): 301–8. http://dx.doi.org/10.1080/01446190500435028.

Lewis, B. 2006. "New Hospital Takes Pulse of Private Investors." *Province*, 13 June.

–. 2008. "New Abbotsford Hospital a Big Step Forward." *Province*, 24 February.

Leyne, L. 2009. "Nanaimo Hopsital Botched C. Difficile Bug Battle, Probe Finds." *Montreal Gazette*, 9 July.

Leys, C. 2010. "Health, Health Care, and Capitalism." *Socialist Register* 46.

Lindgren, A. 2001. "Ontario Health Minister Tony Clement Says No Idea Is Off Limits during the Province's Public Hearings into Medicare Reform." *Postmedia News*, 1 June.

–. 2003. "McGuinty Demands the Premier Halt Public-Private Partnership Hospitals." CanWest News, 26 September.

Local Health Integration Network (LHIN). 2010. *MOHLTC-LHIN Joint Review Framework for Early Capital Planning Stages: Toolkit*. Government of Ontario, 9 November. http://www.centraleastlhin.on.ca/~/media/sites/ce/uploadedfiles/Home_Page/Report_and_Publications/Capital_Planning_Toolkit_-_FINAL_V03__2010-11-09_.pdf.

Loxley, J. 2010. *Public Service, Private Profits*. Fernwood, NS: Black Point.

–. 2012. "Public-Private Partnerships after the Global Financial Crisis: Ideology Trumping Economic Reality." *Studies in Political Economy* 89:7–37.

Loxley, S.J. 1999a. *An Analysis of a Public Private Partnership: The Confederation Bridge*. Ottawa: Canadian Union of Public Employees. 15 May.

–. 1999b. *An Analysis of a Public Private Partnership: The Evergreen Park School, Moncton, New Brunswick*. Ottawa: Canadian Union of Public Employees. 30 March.

Lyons, B.R. 1996. "Empirical Relevance of Efficient Contract Theory: Inter-Firm Contracts." *Oxford Review of Economic Policy* 12 (4): 27–52. http://dx.doi.org/10.1093/oxrep/12.4.27.

Mackenzie, H. 2007. *Doing the Math: Why P3's for Alberta Schools Don't Add Up*. Canadian Union of Public Employees Alberta. http://archive.cupe.ca/updir/cupe_alberta_doing_the_math.pdf.

–. 2009. *Bad Before, Worse Now*. Hugh Mackenzie & Associates. http://www.cupe.bc.ca/sites/default/files/Bad%20Before%20Worse%20Now%20_final_%20_2_.pdf.

Macleod, A. 2007. "Be Our Guest at Public-Private Diners." *Georgia Straight,* 22 February. http://www.straight.com/news/be-our-guest-public-private-diners.

MacPherson, C.B. 1978. *Property: Mainstream and Critical Positions.* Toronto: University of Toronto Press.

Mahon, R. 1977. "Canadian Public Policy: The Unequal Structure of Representation." In Panitch, *Canadian State,* 165–98.

Marx, K. 1977. *Capital,* vol. 1. New York: Vintage Books.

Marx, K., and F. Engels. 1948. *The Communist Manifesto.* New York: International Publishers.

McArthur, G. 2003. "Liberals Would Scrap ROH Deal." *Ottawa Citizen,* 25 September.

McBride, S. 2005. *Paradigm Shift.* 2nd ed. Halifax: Fernwood.

McBride, S., and H. Whiteside. 2011a. "Austerity for Whom?" *Socialist Studies* 7 (1–2): 42–64.

–. 2011b. *Private Affluence, Public Austerity.* Winnipeg: Fernwood.

McDonough, T. 1999. "Gordon's Accumulation Theory: The Highest Stage of Stadial Theory." December. *Review of Radical Political Economics* 31 (4): 6–31. http://dx.doi.org/10.1177/048661349903100402.

–. 2010. "Hospitals Raise Caution over Uniform Pay-for-Performance Rules." *Globe and Mail,* 9 April. http://www.theglobeandmail.com/news/national/hospitals-raise-caution-over-uniform-pay-for-performance-rules/article4260977/.

McFarland, J. 2001. "SuperBuild's Track Record Is No Big Deal." *Globe and Mail,* 15 December.

McInnes, C. 2003. "Proving Ground for a New Way." *Vancouver Sun,* 18 March.

McKellar, J. 2006. "Alternative Delivery Models: The Special Purpose Corporation in Canada." In *Managing Government Property Assets: International Experiences,* ed. O Kaganova and J. McKellar, 335–63. Washington, DC: Urban Institute.

McKenna, B. 2012. "The Hidden Price of Public-Private Partnerships." *Globe and Mail,* 14 October. http://www.theglobeandmail.com/report-on-business/economy/the-hidden-price-of-public-private-partnerships/article4611798/.

McMonagle, D. 1984. "Private Firm May Build Hospital." *Globe and Mail,* 30 June.

McNally, D. 2011. *Global Slump.* Oakland, CA: PM.

Mehra, N. 2005. *Flawed, Failed, Abandoned: 100 P3s, Canadian and International Evidence.* Ontario Health Coalition. http://archive.cupe.ca/updir/Flawed_Failed_Abandoned_-_Final.pdf

Middleton, G. 2002. "Private Sector Will Help Build, Run Hospital Wing." *Province,* 20 October.

Mirza, S. 2007. *Danger Ahead: The Coming Collapse of Canada's Municipal Infrastructure*. Ottawa: Federation of Canadian Municipalities.

Mitchell, B. 1991. "Premier Gets an Earful on Brampton's Cash Woes." *Toronto Star*, 21 February.

Murphy, J. 2007. "Strategic Outsourcing by a Regional Health Authority: The Experience of the Vancouver Island Health Authority." Special issue, *Healthcare Papers* 8:104–11,

Murphy, T. 2008. "The Case for Public-Private Partnerships in Infrastructure." *Canadian Public Administration* 51 (1): 99–126. http://dx.doi.org/10.1111/j.1754-7121.2008.00006.x.

National Audit Office. 2007. *Improving the PFI Tendering Process*. London: NAO.

–. 2012. *Equity Investment in Privately Financed Projects: Report by the Comptroller and Auditor General, February 10*. London: NAO.

"NDP Questions YTG-Partnerships BC Link." 2005. *Whitehorse Star*, 11 August. http://whitehorsestar.com/archive/story/ndp-questions-ytg-partnerships-bc-link/.

New Brunswick Auditor General. 1999. "Chapter 5: Fredericton-Moncton Highway." *Report of the Auditor General*. http://www.gnb.ca/OAG-BVG/1999v1/chap5e.pdf.

North, D.C. 1990. *Institutions, Institutional Change and Economic Performance*. Cambridge: Cambridge University Press. http://dx.doi.org/10.1017/CBO9780511808678.

Northern Health Authority (NHA). 2010. *2010/11–2012/13 Service Plan*. http://www.northernhealth.ca/Portals/0/About/Financial_Accountability/documents/2010-11%20Service%20PLan%20-%20FINAL%20VERSION%20September%202010.pdf.

Nuttall, J. 2012. "Province Fires Cowichan Valley School Board for Passing Deficit." *Globe and Mail*, 2 July. http://www.theglobeandmail.com/news/british-columbia/province-fires-cowichan-valley-school-board-for-passing-deficit/article4385551/.

O'Connor, E. 2004. "Private Sector Admitted to VGH." *Province*, 12 April.

O'Hara, P.A. 1998. "A Social Structure of Accumulation for Long Wave Upswing in Australia?" *Journal of Australian Political Economy* 61:88–111.

–. 2006. *Growth and Development in the Global Political Economy*. London: Routledge.

Ontario Auditor General. 2008. "Brampton Civic Hospital Public-Private Partnership Project." *2008 Annual Report of the Auditor General of Ontario*. http://www.auditor.on.ca/en/reports_en/en08/303en08.pdf.

–. 2010. "Brampton Civic Hospital Public-private Partnerships Project: Follow-up." http://www.auditor.on.ca/en/reports_en/en10/403en10.pdf.

–. 2014. "Infrastructure Ontario – Alternative Financing and Procurement."
   Annual Report of the Auditor General of Ontario. http://www.auditor.
   on.ca/en/reports_en/en14/305en14.pdf.
Ontario Health Coalition (OHC). 2006a. "Bill 36 LHINs Legislation Analysis."
   3 January. http://www.ontariohealthcoalition.ca/wp-content/uploads/
   FULL-REPORT-January-3-2006.pdf.
–. 2006b. "Hamilton Joins More Than 50,000 Ontarians in Saying No to Privatized
   P3 Hospitals." 27 March. http://www.cupe.on.ca/aux_bin.php?auxid=177.
–. 2008. *When Public Relations Trumps Public Accountability: The Evolution of
   Cost Overruns, Service Cuts and Cover-up in the Brampton Hospital P3.* Ontario
   Health Coalition, 7 January. http://www.ontariohealthcoalition.ca/index.
   php/when-public-relations-trumps-public-responsibility/.
"Ontario Health Minister Points to Role of Privatization in Health-Care
   Reform." *Calgary Sun,* 6 September.
Ontario Ministry of Finance. 2009. "Ministry of Energy and Infrastructure –
   The Estimates, 2009–10 – Summary." http://www.fin.gov.on.ca/en/
   budget/estimates/2009-10/volume1/MEI.html.
–. 2012. "Public Sector Salary Disclosure 2012 (Disclosure for 2011):
   Crown Agencies." http://www.fin.gov.on.ca/en/publications/
   salarydisclosure/2012/crown12b.html.
Ontario Ministry of Health. 1996. *A Guide to the Capital Planning Process.*
   Toronto: Queen's Printer. http://www.ontla.on.ca/library/repository/
   mon/23007/193778.pdf.
–. 2011. "Health Infrastructure Renewal Fund Guidelines: Local Health
   Integration Networks." January. Draft.
Ontario Ministry of Infrastructure. 2005. "Five-Year Investment Plan Will Help
   Ensure High-Quality Services for Ontarians." News release, 25 May. http://
   news.ontario.ca/archive/en/2005/05/25/FiveYear-Investment-Plan-will-
   Help-Ensure-HighQuality-Services-for-Ontarians.html.
Ontario Ministry of Municipal Affairs and Housing. 2007. "Amendments to
   Municipal Act, 2001 Proclaimed." News release, 1 January. http://www.
   mah.gov.on.ca/Page1031.aspx
Ontario Ministry of Public Infrastructure Renewal (MPIR). 2004. *Building a
   Better Tomorrow: Infrastructure Planning, Financing and Procurement Framework
   for Ontario's Public Sector.* Toronto: Queen's Printer.
"Ontario Plans First Privately Built Hospital." 2001. *Daily Commercial News and
   Construction Record.* 74 (235).
Ontario Public Service Employees Union (OPSEU). 2007. "Risky Business: The
   Royal Ottawa Mental Health Centre: Ontario's First P3 hospital." *OPSEU
   Local* 479 (June). https://www. opseu.org.

Ontario Standing Committee on Government Agencies. 2008. "Agency Review: Ontario Infrastructure Project Corp. (Infrastructure Ontario)." 17 September. http://www.ontla.on.ca/web/committee-proceedings/committee_transcripts_details.do?locale=en&Date=2008-09-17&ParlCommI D=8859&BillID=&Business=Agency+review%3A+Ontario+Infrastructure+ Projects+Corp.+%28Infrastructure+Ontario%29&DocumentID=23205.

Ontario Standing Committee on Public Accounts. 2009. "2008 Annual Report, Auditor General: Ministry of Energy and Infrastructure, Ministry of Health and Long-Term Care." 25 March. http://www.ontla.on.ca/web/committee-proceedings/committee_transcripts_details.do?locale=en&Date=2009-03-25&ParlCommID=8861&BillID=&Business=2008+Annual+Report% 2C+Auditor+General%3A++Ministry+of+Energy+and+Infrastructure% 2C++Ministry+of+Health+and+Long-Term+Care&DocumentID=23744.

Ontario SuperBuild Corporation. 2000. *Building Ontario's Future: A SuperBuild Progress Report*. December. http://www.fin.gov.on.ca/en/publications/2000/sbfine00.pdf.

Osborne, D., and T. Gaebler. 1992. *Reinventing Government: How the Entrepreneurial Spirit Is Transforming the Public Sector*. Reading: Addison-Wesley.

Palmer, V. 2003. "Community Charter = Hang On to Your Wallet." *Vancouver Sun*, 12 March.

–. 2008. "Premier Shops Around for Expensive Theme." *Vancouver Sun*, 25 September.

Parks, R., and R. Terhart, 2009. *Evaluation of Public-Private Partnerships: Costing and Evaluation Methodology*. Report prepared for the Canadian Union of Public Employees: British Columbia.

Partnerships BC (PBC). n.d. "Projects." http://www.partnershipsbc.ca/files/projects.html.

–. 2004. *Project Report: Achieving Value for Money Academic Ambulatory Care Centre Project*. Victoria: Partnerships BC.

–. 2005. *Project Report: Achieving Value for Money Abbotsford Regional Hospital and Cancer Centre Project*. Victoria: Partnerships BC.

–. 2009. "Fort St John Hospital and Residential Care Project: Financing Structure." 22 July. http://www.partnershipsbc.ca/files/documents/20090722-bg_fsjh-financing-structure-web.pdf.

–. 2010. *2009/2010 Annual Report*. http://www.partnershipsbc.ca/files/documents/partnershipsbc2009-10annualreportfinal.pdf.

–. 2011. *2010/2011 Annual Report*. http://www.partnershipsbc.ca/files/documents/pbc-annualreport-15jun2011.pdf.

Peck, J. 2010. *Constructions of Neoliberal Reason*. Oxford: Oxford University Press. http://dx.doi.org/10.1093/acprof:oso/9780199580576.001.0001.

Peck, J., and A. Tickell. 2002. "Neoliberalizing Space." *Antipode* 34 (3): 380–404. http://dx.doi.org/10.1111/1467-8330.00247.

Pitelis, C. 1992. "Toward a Neo-classical Theory of Institutional Failure." *Journal of Economic Studies* 19 (1). http://dx.doi.org/10.1108/01443589210015926.

Pollock, A., J. Shaoul, and N. Vickers. 2002. "Private Finance and 'Value for Money' in NHS Hospitals: A Policy in Search of a Rationale?" *British Medical Journal* 324:1205–9.

PPP Canada. 2009. *Annual Report 2008–2009*. http://www.p3canada.ca/~/media/english/annual-reports/files/2008-2009%20annual%20report.pdf.

–. 2013. *Water/Wastewater Sector Study*. Ottawa: PPP Canada.

Prahalad, C.K. 2005. *The Fortune at the Bottom of the Pyramid: Eradicating Poverty through Profit and Enabling Dignity and Choice through Markets*. Upper Saddle River, NJ: Wharton School.

"Private Hospital in Abbotsford Opposed by 71 Per Cent of Public, Including Majority of Liberal Supporters: Poll." 2002. Canada Newswire. 7 May.

"Private Hospital Schemes Based on 'Pseudo-Scientific Mumbo-Jumbo,' Warns Britain's Top Financial Watchdog." 2002. Canada Newswire. 26 June.

Project Finance. 2011. "How Bonds Took Over Canada's PPP Market." *Infrastructure Journal and Project Finance Magazine*, 28 November.

Quebec Auditor General. 2009. *Rapport à l'Assemblée nationale pour l'année 2009–2010*. http://www.vgq.gouv.qc.ca/fr/fr_publications/fr_rapport-annuel/fr_2009-2010-T2/fr_Rapport2009-2010-T2-Chap06.pdf.

Rachwalski, M.D., and T. Ross. 2010. "Running a Government's P3 Program: Special Purpose Agency or Line Departments?" June. *Journal of Comparative Policy Analysis* 12 (3): 275–98. http://dx.doi.org/10.1080/13876981003714586.

Reynolds, K. 2011. "How Flipping Equity in P3s Boosts Profits and Ends Up with the Projects Being Run from Channel Islands Tax Havens." *Policy Note*, 9 March. www.policynote.ca/how-flipping-equity-in-p3s-boosts-profits-and-ends-up-with-the-projects-being-run-from-channel-islands-tax-havens/.

–. 2012. "How the Rules Got Fiddled to Make Sure a Public Private Partnership Got Pushed Through." *Policy Note*, 12 July. http://www.policynote.ca/how-the-rules-got-fiddled-to-make-sure-a-public-private-partnership-got-pushed-through/.

Rikowski, G. 2003. "Schools and the GATS Enigma." *Journal for Critical Education Policy Studies* 1:1.

Ronson, J. 2011. "LHINs at Five Years: What Now?" *Longwoods*, 22 June. http://www.longwoods.com/publications/healthcare-policy.

Rouillard, C. 2006. "Public-Private Partnerships and Democratic Governance." Paper presented to the 2006 Canadian Political Science Association's Annual Conference, 1–3 June, York University, Toronto.

The Royal. n.d. *History of the Royal.* http://www.theroyal.ca/about-the-royal/our-history/.

Royal Ottawa Mental Health Centre (ROMHC). 2003. "The Re-development of the Royal Ottawa Hospital: Questions & Answers." 15 September.

Sandborn, T. 2007. "Fraser Health Authority Said No to Private Approach." *Tyee*, 1 February. http://thetyee.ca/News/2007/02/01/FHA/.

–. 2008. "Top Private Health Player in BC Slammed for 'Windfall' Profits." *Tyee*, 12 November. www.thetyee.ca/News/2008/11/12/JohnLaing/.

Sandler, J. 2002. "Large Private Role Eyed for Hospital: Proposed Level of Private Participation in New Abbotsford Hospital Would Be a Canadian First." *Vancouver Sun*, 19 March.

Schliesmann, P. 1997. "Brockville Closing a Lesson for KPH." *Kingston Whig-Standard*, 26 February.

Scott, W.R. 1995. *Institutions and Organizations.* London: Sage.

Selznick, P. 1957. *Leadership in Administration.* New York: Harper & Row.

Shaffer, M. 2006. *The Real Cost of the Sea-to-Sky.* Vancouver: Canadian Centre for Policy Alternatives.

Shaoul, J. 2010. "A Review of Transport Public-Private Partnerships in the UK." In *International Handbook on Public-Private Partnerships*, ed. G.A. Hodge, C. Greve, and A.E. Boardman, 548–67. Cheltenham, UK: Edward Elgar. http://dx.doi.org/10.4337/9781849804691.00034.

Shrybman, S. 2007. "Hospitals and the Principles of Medicare." In *Medicare: Facts, Myths, Problems and Promise*, ed. B. Campbell and G. Marchilden, 197–211. Toronto: James Lorimer.

Siemiatycki, M. 2012. "Is There a Distinctive Canadian PPP Model? Reflections on Twenty Years of Practice." CBS-Sauder-Monash Public-Private Partnership Conference, University of British Columbia, Vancouver.

Siemiatycki, M., and N. Farooqi. 2012. "Value for Money and Risk in Public Private Partnerships." *Journal of the American Planning Association* 78 (3): 286–99. http://dx.doi.org/10.1080/01944363.2012.715525.

Smyth, M. 2001. "Hospital a Good Choice for Privatization Kickoff." *Province*, 21 October.

Smith, P., K. Ginnell, and M. Black. 2010. "Local Governing and Local Democracy in British Columbia." In *British Columbia Politics and Government*, ed. M. Howlett, D. Pilon, and T. Summerville, 245–66. Toronto: Emond Montgomery Publications.

Smith, P., and K. Stewart. 2005. "Local Government Reform in British Columbia, 1991–2005: One Oar in the Water." In *Municipal Reforms in Canada: Dynamics, Dimensions, Determinants*, ed. J. Garcia and E. LeSage, 25–56. Don Mills, ON: Oxford University Press.

Steen, D. 1986. "300-Bed Hospital Proposed for 1993 in Brampton Area." *Toronto Star*, 15 July.

Steffenhagen, J. 2002. "$90 Million Centre Is BC's First Public-Private Partnership." *Vancouver Sun*, 21 October.

Stinson, J., N. Pollak, and M. Cohen. 2005. *The Pains of Privatization*. Vancouver: Canadian Centre for Policy Alternatives.

Sullivan, T., and K. Born. 2011. "LHINs and the Governance of Ontario's Health Care System." Healthy Debate, 29 June. http://healthydebate. ca/2011/06/topic/cost-of-care/lhins-2.

TD Economics. 2004. *Mind the Gap: Finding Money to Upgrade Canada's Aging Public Infrastructure*. Toronto: TD Bank Financial Group.

Tett, G. 2007. "How Monoline Market Works." *Financial Times*, 16 November. http://www.ft.com.

Thornton, E. 2007. "Road to Riches." *Bloomberg Businessweek*, 6 May. http:// www.bloomberg.com.

Tickell, A., and J. Peck. 2003. "Making Global Rules: Globalization or Neoliberalization?" In *Remaking the Global Economy*, ed. J. Peck and H.W-C. Yeung, 163–81. London: Sage.

Timmins, N. 2010. "PFI Projects Hit Fresh Low as Industry Battles to Close Deals." *Financial Times*, 14 January.

Tupper, A., and G.B. Doern, eds. 1981. *Public Corporations and Public Policy in Canada*. Montreal: Institute for Research on Public Policy.

UK Comptroller and Auditor General. 2000. *The Refinancing of the Fazakerley PFI Prison Contract*. London: Stationery Office.

UK Department of Health. 2001. "Press Release, 2001/0553," 16 November.

"Unions Lose Bid to Stop Public-Private Partnerships Involving Ont. Hospitals." 2003. *Daily Commercial News and Construction Record*, 76:189. 6 October.

Van Gramberg, B., and P. Bassett. 2005. *Neoliberalism and the Third Sector in Australia*. Working Paper Series, No. 5. Melbourne: Victoria University. School of Management.

Vancouver Coastal Health (VCHA). n.d. "Board Members." http://www.vch.ca/ about_us/leadership/board_of_directors/board_members/.

–. 2010. *2010/11–2012/13 Service Plan*. http://www.vch.ca/media/health_ service_plan2011_13.pdf.

Vancouver Island Health Authority (VIHA). 2010. *VIHA 2010/11–2012/13 Service Plan*. http://www.viha.ca/NR/rdonlyres/AADEEF61-F0F4-47F8-B65B-268D2F6D1FDB/0/HSP_2008_2009.pdf.

Vining, A., and A.E. Boardman. 2008. "Public-Private Partnerships in Canada: Theory and Evidence." *Canadian Public Administration* 51 (1): 9–44. http:// dx.doi.org/10.1111/j.1754-7121.2008.00003.x.

Wall, A., and C. Connolly. 2009. "The Private Finance Initiative." *Public Management Review* 11 (5): 707–24. http://dx.doi. org/10.1080/14719030902798172.

Waterston, L. 2012. "The Future of PPP Financing." Presentation to EPEC Private Sector Forum, "Financing Future Infrastructure," 6 June, Brussels. http://www.eib.org/epec/resources/presentations/psf-06062012-presentation-smbc.pdf.

"'Wealth Equals Health,' Canadian Doctors Say: Lower Income Groups Report Poorer Health." 2012. CBC News, 13 August. http://www.cbc.ca/news/health/wealth-equals-health-canadian-doctors-say-1.1178526.

Whiteside, H. 2012. "Crises of Capital and the Logic of Dispossession and Repossession." *Studies in Political Economy* 89:59–78.

Whitfield, D. 2005. "Building Schools for Shareholders." *Red Pepper*.

–. 2006. "The Marketisation of Teaching." *PFI Journal* 52:92–3.

–. 2009. "Profiteering from Public Private Partnerships." *Guardian*, 10 December. www.guardianpublic.co.uk/ppp-projects-investment-funds.

–. 2010. *The Global Auction of Public Assets: Public Sector Alternatives to the Infrastructure Market and Public Private Partnerships*. Nottingham, UK: Spokesman.

–. 2011. *The £10bn Sale of Shares in PPP Companies: New Source of Profits for Builders and Banks*. European Services Strategy Unit. http://www.european-services-strategy.org.uk/outsourcing-ppp-library/pfi-ppp/the-ps10bn-sale-of-shares-in-ppp-companies-new/10bn-sale-of-ppp-shares.pdf.

"William Osler Health Centre, Etobicoke Hospital Campus." 2002. Canada Newswire, 13 March.

Wolfe, D. 1977. "The State and Economic Policy in Canada, 1968–1975." In *The Canadian State: Political Economy and Political Power*, ed. Leo Panitch, 251–88. Toronto: University of Toronto Press.

Wood, E.M. 1981. "The Separation of the Economic and the Political in Capitalism." *New Left Review* 127 (May–June), 66–95.

Index

Studies in Comparative Political Economy and Public Policy